About the Authors:

Gwendolyn D. Scott, who has previously authored several Health Education texts, is presently Director of the Health Education Curriculum Center at Kent State University. She is Professor Emeritus from that same institution and has consultant positions with Community Health Agencies, the public school system, and the Ohio Department of Education. She also directs Teacher Inservice Workshops, an experience that is reflected strongly in this text.

Mona W. Carlo is also an experienced author in the field of Health Education. She participates actively in numerous Health and Education associations and is president of the Northeast Ohio Health Education Association. She is consultant for Public School Health Education and Community Health Agencies as well as director of Teacher Inservice Workshops. She presently teaches Health Education for the Berea City School District in Ohio.

Both authors have multi-level teaching experience which they have condensed and organized effectively here into a practical handbook on Elementary Health Education: LEARNING — FEELING — DOING.

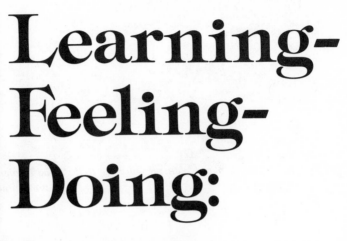

Learning-Feeling-Doing:

designing creative learning experiences for elementary health education

GWENDOLYN D. SCOTT, Ed.D

MONA W. CARLO, M.Ed.

PRENTICE-HALL, INC.
Englewood Cliffs, N.J. 07632

Library of Congress Cataloging in Publication Data

Scott, Gwendolyn D
  Learning — feeling — doing.

  Includes bibliographical references.
  1. Health education (Elementary) I. Carlo,
Mona W., joint author. II. Title.
LB1587.A3S36   372.3'7   78-9331
ISBN 0-13-527689-6

You don't have to plan to fail; all you have to do is fail to plan.
Anonymous

Printed in the United States of America
10 9 8 7 6 5 4 3 2 1

Prentice-Hall International, Inc., *London*
Prentice-Hall of Australia Pty. Limited, *Sydney*
Prentice-Hall of Canada, Ltd., *Toronto*
Prentice-Hall of India Private Limited, *New Delhi*
Prentice-Hall of Japan, Inc., *Tokyo*
Prentice-Hall of Southeast Asia Pte. Ltd., *Singapore*
Whitehall Books Limited, *Wellington, New Zealand*

Acknowledgements

We would like to recognize a group of professional people, craftsmen all, who were concerned enough about the art of growing to share their skills and creativity to help achieve the aim of this book.

To Elaine Seidenwand and Dawn Hilston, former students with exceptional talent, we are particularly grateful. Both shared their creative writing skills in the development of sample learning experiences in entire concepts.

When artistic talent and support were needed, Laurel Wilcox of Kent State University and Earle Ziska of Middleburg Heights Junior High School cared and shared.

Mollie Carlo Wilson, a creative elementary school teacher, recognized the need and provided the incentive for the development of stories to introduce the concepts.

When the idea of using a song in a learning activity seemed appropriate, we supplied the lyrics, Don Masaitis and Barbara Morrow composed the music, and Berda Allen did the arrangement.

Our typist, Connie Spees, took time after her normal job responsibilities, to take on our project and meet our needs.

To the many others who are noted in the body of the book we extend our heartfelt appreciation for allowing us to use their ideas. We learn so much from our students and participants.

G.D.S. and *M.W.C.*

Illustrations

CONCEPT 11

contents

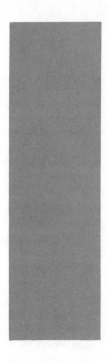

CONCEPT 5: There are Reciprocal Relationships Involving Man, Disease and Environment **133**

CONCEPT 6: The Family Serves to Perpetuate Man and Fulfill Certain Health Needs **155**

CONCEPT 7: Personal Health Practices are Affected by a Complexity of Forces, Often Conflicting **175**

CONCEPT 8: Utilization of Health Information, Products and Services is Guided by Values and Perceptions **196**

preface

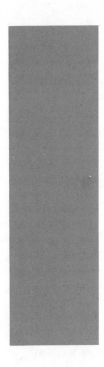

Dear Colleague,

At some point in your professional education there came a realization that life is guided by knowledge, drives, emotions, attitudes, experiences and human relationships. Have you also recognized that each of these motivators is an integral dimension in health education? They all deal directly with the learner as a *total person* facing exciting new experiences from moment to moment.

By the time a child enters the school scene, he/she is already bombarded with accurate or inaccurate health information fed to him by the example of others via verbal and non-verbal communication. By this time the learner's own health behaviors and attitudes toward health are fairly set in the mold. Good or bad, the child tends to imitate the behaviors of the adults who are significant in his/her life. This is not to say that these attitudes and behaviors are permanent or unchangeable. "Change" is what education is all about—*change that improves the quality of life in every way!* As you accept this neophyte learner into your sphere of influence, your role as a compassionate, humanistic, well-prepared facilitator of learning is of immeasurable importance. You are one of the *significant adults* in this child's life! It is your responsibility to provide experiences which may serve as catalysts in helping each learner to become self-motivated. The goal toward which we all are working is to encourage our students to make decisions that will enhance his/her growing and developing process—a heavy burden, admittedly.

You, as a "pre" or practicing professional have already indicated that you *are* a "caring" person simply because you are reading this. You are seeking professional growth.

You may have had little or no preparation in the field of health education. Your teaching certificate may indicate a variety of disciplines you are qualified to teach, but it may nowhere list health education as being one. The fact remains that you, and EVERY TEACHER IS A HEALTH EDUCATOR, directly or indirectly. If you have but partially recognized this fact and have made only a slight pass at including health education in your everyday teaching, think seriously about including it now. Using health information in your particular area of expertise can not only augment your teaching in that discipline, but can also add a new dimension to the total health education experience of each of your students. The student may come to recognize that health education is not an isolated offering, but rather it is an integral part of all learning and living. By its very nature, health education is *education in the skills of living.*

Those of you who are practicing professional health educators realize that health education is dynamic. The areas of emphases are constantly changing as man solves some of the old problems that have plagued him, and creates new ones that arise because of the abuse of his body and his environment.

Each person begins very early in life to make decisions that affect the status of personal health. At first the decisions are at a relatively unconscious level—i.e., refusing foods offered or spitting them out. Gradually, decisions are made at a conscious level—on the basis of "I want," "I like," "I won't," or "I will."

The knowledge of health and the understanding of human behavior has the potential for providing the student with a more rational basis for decision-making. As a result of the increasing emphasis on these two components of health, there has been a drastic change in the instructional aspects of health education.

It is becoming more rare for the student to be receiving anatomy and physiology under the aegis of health education. Rather, these areas are being rightly assigned to the biological sciences.

With the changes occurring in the classrooms, we see student interest growing as they become involved in experiences that have meaning in their daily lives.

The dynamics of health education are encompassed in understanding human behavior (its causes and consequences), and particularly behaviors that affect the student's own health and that of the community of mankind. *How you, as a facilitator of learning, provide experiences for this kind of understanding is pivotal.* It is hoped that this book will be helpful to you in your efforts.

As a "significant person" in the lives of others, you probably already recognize:

1. that the development of concepts of healthful living permeates every educational endeavor;
2. that community and world health depend upon individual behaviors and attitudes;
3. that health behaviors can be changed; and,
4. that there is *no* discipline that offers more opportunity for *Learning, Feeling,* and *Doing* activities applicable to everyday living than those available in health education.

Because you *are* so influential in nurturing others, we wish to "wave the flag" vigorously and urge each of you to "make health education your bag"—now, more than ever!

Sincerely,

Gwen and Mona

introduction: put a dinger in your bell

You have either chosen to become a health educator or health education itself is an area of responsibility within your teaching. How lucky you are! There is no subject more dynamic, more exciting, or more relevant to every living person than one's own health. The question is: How can you accept this feeling of super-importance yourself, and in turn project it to the kids you teach? You have a beautiful bell — how do you ring it?

It's true that there is no magic wand that can be waved, or no tune that can be played in anyone's class that will cause every student to be totally committed to the learning. But it is a certainty that . . .

    . . . if you are not turned on,

    . . . if you do not *really* know *each* of your students and understand his or her uniqueness,

    . . . if you do not consider this uniqueness in your planning,

    . . . if the goals you set and the objectives you design are focused on your performance rather than your students',

    . . . if you limit student involvement in both the learning and evaluative process,

    . . . if you are succeeding in stifling your own creativity by failing to use and adapt ideas from others to meet the needs and interests of your kids,

... if your philosophy and your teaching do not reflect a beautiful blending of *Learning* and *Feeling* and *Doing*, ...

then very little is going to happen in your classroom that will cause more than loud yawns, boredom, and/or disruptive behavior.

It is the fervent hope of the authors that this book will spur your interest in helping health education become one of the most successful experiences in the school life of your students. We are offering you ideas, but you must ring the bell!

This is one of a series of books that responds to the types of assistance requested by teachers to facilitate their instruction. Namely, these types are: (1) assistance in applying the causal behavioral approach to health education; (2) assistance in utilizing behavioral objectives; (3) assistance in using values clarification techniques in health education; (4) assistance in designing learning experiences that involve students and emphasize the affective and psychomotor domains of learning; (5) assistance in having examples of learning experiences that have been designed by others; (6) assistance in adapting others' ideas to the needs of their students. If these are *your* needs, fellow educator, read on!

Panacea? No! Recipe book? No! Encouragement, suggestions, ideas, tried and proven-in-the-classroom strategies and learning experiences? Yes! Our goal and your goal are identical — to improve health education for our kids so that the behaviors they choose will enable them to live more fully. It is then that your bell will become a bell instead of a hunk of metal. You are the dinger — you make the difference!

expecting with understanding

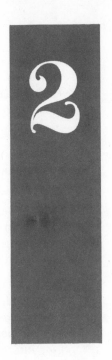

Yes, Virginia, Everyone is Unique

How many times in their academic experiences do teachers have the concept of "individual differences" impressed upon them? It would be a rarity if anyone in education could not expound at length on the meaning of this phrase or its derivatives — "no two people are alike," "each individual is unique," and so on. The concept is beautiful and true. It is basic to the tenets of democracy and educators accept it completely — in theory. How unfortunate that more of them do not utilize the concept in practice — in their everyday teaching! They talk a good game, but playing that game is something else. If the concept is true, then why do so many professionals at all levels indicate by their behavior that they are actually envisioning the class as a unified structure rather than a collection of unique individuals? It is not a rare occurrence for classes to be taught as though all students:

— have identical needs
— come from the same type of family background
— have had similar past experiences
— hold the same personal values

—should accept for themselves the values of the teachers

—having reached the chronological age for the grade level, automatically possess the skills required for success

The Clout of Verbal and Nonverbal Behavior

There are verbal and nonverbal teacher behaviors both in and out of the classroom that project these ideas to students, to other teachers, and to observers. In the classroom, it's not uncommon to hear these comments or to observe these actions:

"Jerry, you shouldn't feel that way."

"Very good, George. It always pays to be . . . (kind, honest, good, etc.)."

"Sherry, you shouldn't act that way. You're _____ years old and not a baby any more."

"No, Rita, you're wrong to have that attitude about it. The right way is . . ."

"Fathers and mothers love their children."

"Jack, if you continue to act like a first grader, I can make arrangements for you to spend the rest of the day with the first graders."

Notice the smiles, the nods of approval, the hugs, the frowns, the tightened lips, the shakes of the head that effectively convey to the student how either his action or his comment is being received. It may be an oversimplified generalization, but the constant bombardment of clues such as these tend to be very reinforcing to students. When the feedback received is of a positive nature, the student learns to discuss his ideas and to express his attitudes. When the feedback is negative, the student learns to play a passive role in the classroom. The message comes through loud and clear that to be "successful" in the educational system and not be "put down" by the teacher, he or she must avoid expressing real attitudes, challenging the teacher's ideas, or displaying feelings. The enthusiasm and honesty that is so freely expressed by youngsters in the primary grades is gradually extinguished. We end up playing a significant role in turning off the joys of learning for many students when our goal is the exact opposite. So we return to the original question: Why do so many professionals deal with their students as a collective whole rather than as individuals who are both unique and capable?

Facilitator, Heal Thyself!

Since teachers are also unique, no one reason is applicable to all. Rather, there are several probable explanations that contribute to the problem. Typical teacher comments can again provide clues to the reasons for teacher behavior.

> "I don't know about parents these days. My kids just don't seem to have any values."

Everyone has "values." What is so often unrecognized is that what a student values or prizes is often different from what the teacher values. Teachers tend to have a mental model of the "ideal" student — one who is interested, energetic, respectful, self-motivated, helpful, honest, truthful, considerate, clean, mature, and well-behaved. When a student fails — as he will — to fit into this preconceived mold, judgments are made, and both the student and the teacher demonstrate their respective frustration by altered behavior.

Teachers begin to rationalize their behavior to themselves and others by thinking and saying such things as:

> "What am I supposed to do? I have wall-to-wall kids. If those administrators . . ."
>
> "It's the parents' fault for not instilling values in their kids."
>
> "The kids' behavior is getting worse every year! I sent five to the office from one class yesterday."

It is so very comforting to use as scapegoats the school administration, the students, or their parents. When we can put the blame on others, we don't have to examine the possibility that our own behavior could be contributing to the problems that we see in the classroom.

> "With all of the subjects I teach in a day, it's utterly unrealistic to expect me to prepare materials for different learning levels in each."

This comment sounds so logical that some teachers are convinced that it just isn't possible to provide different experiences in their classes. Thus, these teachers can settle comfortably in their complacency and mouth the same generalization for maintaining the status quo.

Stop and think for a moment. Is there really anything unique about planning for different levels? Teachers in the one-room school did it. Teachers with groupings of "Bluebirds," "Redbirds," and "Yellowbirds," did it.

Teachers today are doing it when they see the advantages that accrue.

Consider the following:

1. When students are involved and successful in their learning, teachers in turn feel successful and enjoy their teaching.
2. Changes in teacher behavior promote changes in student behavior.
3. Reducing the frustration of the students pays off in the reduction of frustration of the teacher.
4. If teachers can bring themselves to ask, "What am I doing that is causing these behaviors?" they can identify ways to modify their own behavior.

All of these concepts scream out the fact that higher expectations of learning, feeling, and doing can be a reality if teachers will genuinely recognize that students *are* at different points in the growth and development continuum, and that as teachers they must play a leading role in helping each child's advancement.

It is perfectly obvious to all elementary teachers that students have a wide ability range in reading skills. But is it as obvious that reading practice and improvement must not be confined to reading class? Is there a single, valid reason why teachers cannot design lessons in health education (or any other subject area) that recognize reading ability variances and build in opportunities for students to enrich their skills? Everyone needs to remember that "reading," as a subject in the curriculum, has no content as such. The content is found in everything the child reads—including health education materials.

To have high expectations for student performance in health education is not idealistic or visionary. The key to the puzzle lies in the acceptance of each student for what he is as a person and then in providing for his particular growth needs. This is "expecting with understanding."

behavior
is for real

The Mission

As facilitators of health education, your real mission is to help students to understand and modify their health behaviors so they can improve the quality of their living. It does not suffice for them to learn only the facts concerned with health. Content *is* extremely important as a basis for decision-making. But content alone is not the living end. Everyone must deal with his own behavior and that of others every conscious moment of his life. Therefore, in order for a program of health education to approach its potential, the teacher must skillfully blend all facets together.

Students must be provided with a variety of opportunities: opportunities to examine their present values, opportunities to learn factual information that may encourage them to reexamine those values, opportunities to solve hypothetical problems that are within their realm of experience, opportunities to understand reasons for their own behavior as well as for the behavior of others. To *change* or to *deal* with changes in health behaviors, both you and your students need to have some insight into the nature of behavior.

What Is Behavior?

Human behavior is very complex. Yet the basic concepts of behavior can be understood by almost any school-age child without getting into the heavy stuff. And you, the facilitator, don't need to be a trained psychologist to teach toward an understanding of concepts at their level of understanding. The first step in accomplishing this is to have a working definition for the word "behavior." Behavior is an *observable* act performed in response to internal and/or external stimuli. The word *observable* is extremely important in differentiating between a behavior and a nonbehavior. In order to be a behavior, the act must be something that can be seen, heard, physically felt, or measured. A nonbehavior is a process that takes place internally — such as thinking, understanding, or feeling emotionally. These nonbehaviors cannot be observed because they take place within a person. However, the *results* or *expressions* of nonbehaviors *are* behaviors because they are observable. Examples:

sadness (NB) --→ crying (B)
understanding (NB) --→ explaining (B)
thinking (NB) --→ expressing (B)
happiness (NB) --→ smiling (B)
nervousness (NB) --→ fidgeting (B)

The basic concepts of behavior can be stated in this way:

1. Behavior is caused.
2. Behavior has a field of alternatives from which to choose.
3. Behavior has consequences (effects, results).
4. Behavior may be judged "good" or "bad" depending upon the values of the people affected by it.
5. Behavior can be changed.

BEHAVIORS HAVE CAUSES

Behaviors enable a person to reach desired goals. What the goals are, are determined by needs. (NEEDS is the big word). All human beings have basic needs that must be met in order for growth and development to take place. It is not always an easy task to fulfill basic needs. When they are not satisfied or they are blocked, behavior changes in order to compensate for them. The needs a person has are dictated by the total of his/her life experiences up to the present moment.

Maslow[1] indicated five basic needs that all humans have. In

[1] A.H. Maslow, "A Theory of Human Motivation," *Psychological Review*, 1943, 50, 370-96.

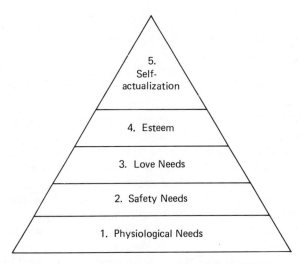

Figure 1-1. Maslow's Hierarchy of Basic Needs

classifying them from most important to least important, a hierarchy
of needs develops.

1. *Physiological Needs* (the need for food, water, shelter, warmth, exercise, rest)
2. *Safety Needs* (the need to be safe from harm)
3. *Love Needs* (the need to love and be loved, to need and be needed)
4. *Esteem Needs* (the need to feel worthwhile, important, accepted, appreciated, and to have self-respect)
5. *Self-actualization* (the need to become the person one is capable of being)

People have many lesser needs, but all can be classified into this
hierarchy. Physiological needs, of course, are the most basic of all,
for without those being satisfied the life processes could not proceed.
Each of the other needs in the hierarchy is built upon this base, and
they evolve upward in order of their importance. But a person will
give up all of these to satisfy his basic physical needs. Once the
physical needs are secured, he is able to reach upward to protect and
preserve his life, to participate in the continuation of the race, to
satisfy his acceptance needs, and to fulfill the potential qualities that
enable life to become a more fulfilling experience, to himself or
herself as well as to others.

Behaviors reflect needs being acted out. But needs alone are not
the only ingredient that dictate which behavior from a field of alternatives will be chosen to be performed. There are two other stars in

9

the play that specifically influence this selection of behavior. One is a person's immediate physical setting — that is, where and with whom the person is at any given moment. The other is the knowledge the person has about himself or herself — the past experiences, the values, the human relationships, the goals, the skills, the ideas, and the present attitudes.

The setting in which a person is operating, along with the other people present, exert physical, emotional, and social pressures that heavily prejudice that person's behavior choice. Something that he/she might never think of doing under other circumstances, he/she may now choose to do because of where and with whom he/she finds himself or herself. Perhaps this kind of super-influence is most noticeable in the lives of young people who are so vulnerable to peer pressures and conformity. But they don't own it — we all act under these conditions.

Knowledge of self also tends to be a very substantial motivation in a person's choice of a behavior. If an individual has experienced the results of a like-behavior before, he or she can reasonably assume what will happen if it is repeated. If the results satisfied his/her needs, then the behavior pattern will be reinforced, especially if the place and the people involved are the same. If the results were unsatisfactory, the person may deem it wise to choose an alternate behavior because of the frustration that may have been experienced.

Behavior, then, is caused by the interaction of needs, immediate physical setting, and knowledge of self. Even though the majority of the time the chosen behavior is performed spontaneously, nonetheless, all three components play an active role in its selection. When these factors are put into equation form and explained, it is relatively easy for students to understand.

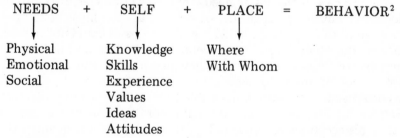

NEEDS   +   SELF   +   PLACE   =   BEHAVIOR[2]

Physical	Knowledge	Where
Emotional	Skills	With Whom
Social	Experience	
	Values	
	Ideas	
	Attitudes	

Allow your students to analyze a given list of behaviors by sug-

---

[2] *Dealing With Aggressive Behavior — A Curriculum for Middle School and Junior High School.* (Student Book). A Title III ESEA Project Granted by the Division of Research, Planning, and Development, Ohio Department of Education. Printed by Educational Research Council of America, 1971, p. 17.

gesting what needs, knowledge of self, and environments may have interacted to make each behavior occur. Examples:

> Dana and Jackie stole several items from the discount store.
>
> Jamie brushes her teeth every day.
>
> Kim sneaks away with friends to smoke.
>
> Robbie throws spitballs in class.
>
> Bill dresses warmly because he must walk a long distance to school.
>
> John looks both ways before crossing the street.
>
> Gail picks on smaller kids while playing on the playground.
>
> Jim does many chores to help out at home.

These are only a few suggestions. Make a list of behaviors suitable to your students in your environment and at their age level.

BEHAVIORS HAVE ALTERNATIVES

Rarely does someone set out to reach a desired goal and find that there is smooth sailing. More often than not the road is quite bumpy. There may be detours or even barriers that may stop the progress completely. These obstructions to fulfilling needs are frustrations. Everyone experiences frustrations and *must* deal with them. Sometimes frustrations are self-created by the behavior a person chooses to employ. Other times the frustrations may be set up by the behavior of others or by a person's own biological limitations. Whatever the cause, when frustration does rear its ugly head a person can either:

> 1. accept it as a challenge to overcome, or
> 2. accept it as a failure to brood over, ignore, or simply hide from.

If the person accepts it as being a challenge, he/she will seek to devise alternative means to reach his/her desired outcome, testing each to see if it might be successful. If it is successful, then the behavior is reinforced. If he/she does not deal with the frustration and continually accepts defeat, his/her self-image diminishes. In either case, behavior changes.

All of this is a rather lengthy way of saying:

> 1. there are alternative behaviors that can be selected for every situation,
> 2. everyone needs to develop skills for coping with the inevitable frustrations which will arise,
> 3. frustrations in fulfilling needs lead to alternative behaviors, and
> 4. alternative behaviors may be of an "adjusting" nature or "maladjusting" nature, depending upon whether the need has been satisfied or merely glossed over superficially.

The choice of which behavior, from the field of alternatives, is to be performed is determined by the needs, the environment, and the sum total of past experiences. The behavioral equation now appears as:

$$\text{NEEDS} \quad + \quad \text{SELF} \quad + \quad \text{PLACE} \quad = \quad \text{BEHAVIOR}$$
$$\downarrow$$
$$\text{ALTERNATIVES}$$

BEHAVIORS HAVE CONSEQUENCES

In nature, there is a universal law that states that for every action there is a reaction. This law also holds true for behavior. Behavior is the *action* that results from the *interaction* of internal and external stimuli on a person. What happens as a result of the behavior is the *reaction* consequence of the behavior.

Consequences:

1. can be physical, mental, emotional, social, or any combination of these in nature; and
2. can be immediate (they happen right away) or long-range (they happen some time in the future).

An example:

Kim sneaks away with friends to smoke.

Immediate Physical Effects (Possible)

1. The central nervous system is stimulated
2. There is a tobacco odor on his/her person
3. The group is discovered by an authority figure and punished
4. They are not discovered

Long-range Physical Effects (Possible)

1. Smoking can cause a physical dependency
2. Chance of chronic cough, lung cancer, heart involvement, and/or emphysema at an earlier age

Immediate Mental Effects (Possible)

1. "Sneaking" indicates that the group is fleeing from reality
2. Getting away with the behavior may reinforce it

Long-range Mental Effects (Possible)

1. Smoking can become habitual
2. A psychological dependency may result
3. Defiance of other rules and/or authority figures may result

Immediate Emotional Effects (Possible)

1. Thrill, excitement of doing something against the rules and getting away with it
2. Worry and anxiety if caught
3. Feeling important and grown-up
4. Feeling apprehensive

Long-range Emotional Effects (Possible)

1. Breaking other rules for kicks
2. Performing other behaviors to satisfy emotional needs (eating, drinking, etc.)

Immediate Social Effects (Possible)

1. Acceptance by friends
2. Looking big and important to others
3. Strained relationships with authority figures
4. Rejection by some classmates

Long-range Social Effects (Possible)

1. Setting a poor example for younger people
2. Air-polluter
3. Bad breath may inhibit social interaction
4. Illness may force dependence upon others (society, family)

Some of these items listed may seem far-fetched, but remember, they are only examples of possible effects. Kids may be able to come up with many more consequences.

Consequences of behavior will determine, to a great extent, if the behavior will be repeated or if there will be experimentation with an alternative behavior to reach a desired outcome.

The behavioral equation is now complete and looks like this:

NEEDS + SELF + PLACE

= BEHAVIOR ⟶ CONSEQUENCES

ALTERNATIVES *IMMEDIATE* *LONG-RANGE*

IMMEDIATE	*LONG-RANGE*
Physical	Physical
Mental	Mental
Emotional	Emotional
Social	Social

BEHAVIOR MAY BE "GOOD" OR "BAD"

Dana and Jackie stole several items from the discount store.

This is merely an example of a behavior that some kids may have chosen to perform. It is also a good situation to illustrate that the behavior may be judged as "good" or "bad" dependent upon the values of the people affected by it.

If Dana and Jackie get away with the act they may judge it to be an expedient way to obtain material possessions. The behavior may also enable each one to be admired by the other, or by others in their peer group. In addition, it may also fulfill their needs for thrills, excitement, new experiences, and being successful. The store owner, on the other hand, more than likely will view this as a very destructive behavior because of the cost of the merchandise he has lost. Society in general sees this activity as a crime for which it must pay in the form of higher prices.

If Jackie and Dana are caught in the act of shoplifting, they may change their attitude about it being a good behavior because of the consequences they might face.

Parents may or may not judge the behavior as good or bad, depending upon their value system. Some would judge it bad only if the kids were caught, because the behavior would reflect upon them. Even if the kids were not apprehended and the parents discovered in some other way that their children had committed the crime, they might judge it to be "bad" and do something to halt this kind of activity.

This same kind of analysis can be applied to any other kind of behavior. Try it with this example of a health behavior:

"Jamie brushes her teeth every day."

How might these people judge this behavior?

1. Jamie
2. Parents
3. Peers
4. Dentist

You will find that your students are very capable of performing this type of analysis and understanding that values affect judgment.

BEHAVIOR CAN BE CHANGED

All behavior can be changed — those that are constructive in the eye of the performer can be turned into those that he/she judges to be destructive. Conversely, those the performer views as destructive can be turned into behaviors he/she sees as constructive.

You have probably concluded by now that there are many factors that "play" on changes of behavior. Some of these may be:

1. an adjustment of needs and goals
2. additional life experiences
3. frustrations and successes
4. self-concept
5. external and internal motivations,
6. biological limitations or potentials

The fact remains that behavior can be changed and it is multi-determined. It is not the purpose of this chapter to delve deeper into the study of human behavior but only to suggest that, in order to bring about changes in behavior, a basic understanding of the subject is necessary for students as well teachers. In essence, behavioral changes occur as the person places a different value on any of the various factors that make up the behavior itself.

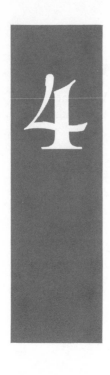

4 get off the stage and into the groove

Desks Aren't for Hiding Behind

What is a desk? The dictionary describes it as a table equipped with drawers and/or compartments with a top for writing, drawing, or reading. Desks are very useful pieces of furniture. As teachers, we learn to expect our classrooms to come equipped with student desks as well as a teacher's desk. How often, though, do we consider to what use these desks are put?

Let's look at the desks in a self-contained classroom. As we look at student and teacher desks, we find that both are used to store books and other materials as well as to hold materials for reading, writing, or drawing. In many classrooms the teacher's desk is in the center front with the student desks in neat, formal rows facing the teacher's desk. In other rooms small tables replace the student desks, but again the formal placement is the most common, with students seated on the far side of the table so that they all face the teacher.

Although there is no conclusive evidence, we would suggest that the primary reason for the formal arrangements in most classrooms at every level is historical. Until the 1930s, manufacturers made student desks so that they had to be immobilized by permanently screwing them into wooden runners. Thus, the desks were as much a part of the permanent building as the placement of the windows or the chalkboards.

Since then, the free-standing desk or tablet arm chair has been developed, and yet customs change slowly. Generations of teachers and custodians "know" that the proper organization of a classroom entails putting the chairs or desks in nice, neat rows.

Consider what this formal arrangement tends to foster. The students are facing the teacher's desk with an excellent view of the various hairstyles of their classmates. They have limited opportunities to have eye contact with each other. The central location of the teacher's desk encourages teachers to use their desk as a pulpit from which to expound, a protective device to hide behind, or a perch upon which to sit. It also provides a natural barrier between the "receivers" and the "giver." Thus, the students are encouraged to remain passive receivers while the teacher becomes the active participant.

What's so important about changing the arrangement of a classroom? Nothing, if you are satisfied with the status quo — satisfied with a placement of furniture that nonverbally shouts, "I am the leader — you are the follower! I am the keeper of the 'pearls of wisdom' which I shall dole out to you, one by one." But if you wish to set a tone to bring about a comfortable interaction between students as well as between you and your students, consider periodically rearranging the classroom.

Survey your room for an obscure corner. Consider moving your filing cabinet, desk, and perhaps a small table into that section to provide yourself with an area that is semi-private. Here it is possible to arrange materials for future classes on the table, keep the materials filed that aren't presently being used, and provide a working area for the times you aren't actively involved in facilitating learning. Students have no difficulty in accepting that portion of the room as being "off-limits" to them.

Whether the desk is in the front or the back isn't particularly important, but placing it in an out-of-the-way area will reduce the probability of the teacher overusing it as an anchor.

What can be done with the student desks or tables? The type of learning experiences that are planned will often dictate this. For example, learning stations using audiovisual equipment at several stations mandates the placement of tables around the perimeter of the room near the electrical outlets. This arrangement would only be logical for the period of time allotted to station learning.

For a basic arrangement, consider one of the following suggestions. Each of these arrangements makes it easy for students to interact with other students as well as to see the chalkboard or the screen which is usually mounted either center front or in a front corner.

One of the most effective basic arrangements is to make a double-rowed horseshoe with the open end on the chalkboard side. With this arrangement, chairs or desks can easily be rearranged for small group work. Floor space is available for role playing, skits, or values activities. The teacher–facilitator can sit with the students for discussions or move with ease from one group to another. Space is also provided for a table to be moved into the open area that contains reference materials needed for the learning experiences. A modification of this is the three-sided rectangle two rows deep.

Another basic arrangement particularly useful in rooms without windows or in rooms without excessive glare is one placing three rows on one side of the room facing a similar three rows on the opposite side.

Rectangular tables, when placed around the perimeter of the room, make very serviceable learning stations for continuous progress learning or audio–tutorial learning experiences. Tables also facilitate interpersonal interaction for small group projects.

For total class involvement, it is more difficult to work with tables. If the class is small, the tables can be placed in a hollow square formation with the open end toward the screen or chalkboard. The students are then seated on the outside facing in. When the size of the class necessitates seating on both sides of the table, there is really no efficient formation that will eliminate a large number of students having their backs toward other students.

If it can be arranged with the custodian, student desks supplemented by two or three tables provides ideal classroom flexibility.

Of course, the placement of the furniture within the room is only one facet in setting an atmosphere conducive to learning. The single most important individual in any classroom is the teacher. She or he is being paid to facilitate the educational achievement for all of the assigned students. As such, the teacher is responsible for carefully selecting the concepts, skillfully designing the learning objectives, and proficiently planning the learning experiences that will motivate students to become involved in their own education.

The physical atmosphere of the classroom can be used to help the students get the feeling that the teacher is "with them" and not "over them." Moreover, students find it is intriguing when a variety of arrangements are employed with their desks. Desks are not for hiding behind — for students as well as for teachers!

A Moving Target is Hard to Hit

Being a successful facilitator of learning takes an abundance of both mental and physical energy. Dealing day after day with the everpresent challenges from within the classroom as well as without is extremely demanding. In this book the "without" pressures will not be dealt with. Rather, the focus throughout is on what takes place "within the room," and *that* is certainly exacting enough.

Earlier in this book the clout of nonverbal teacher behaviors was discussed. It is appropriate now to deal with one more aspect of this, and that is the mobility or immobility of the teacher in the room.

Movement demands energy. Inaction conserves energy. Sometimes it is expedient to be semi-static, but more times than not, teacher mobility in combination with teacher effervescence can be a positive motivating force in the classroom. Students tend to respond to action with activity on their part. Conversely, a sedentary, fixed teacher (especially one fixed behind a desk) can rightfully expect the same kind of reaction from the kids.

Move! Even in an ordinary classroom discussion, change position. It keeps the students alert. It demands, at least, that they must move their eyes. During group or individual learning activity, move about. Take the opportunity to give attention to all students, to compliment them, to criticize constructively, to touch. Grade papers some other time. The critical time in learning is while it is taking place.

Yes, mobility involves the spending of energy, but the results may be worth it.

Discovering the Big Idea

The ultimate aim in any educational endeavor is for the learner, whatever his status in life, to learn. Ultimately, the major responsibility for the attainment of this goal seems to rest squarely on the shoulders of the teacher. The teacher is the key — the buck stops here. At times this responsibility seems overwhelming, but a combination of guts, persistence, endurance, a sense of humor, and experience help every teacher to travel the rocky road a little more smoothly.

It takes guts to initiate change in teaching style when it seems appropriate to do so. When something "bombs," persistence and endurance are needed in order for the teacher to shift gears and take off in another direction. Let's face it, "bombs" are not all that bad, especially if the "bomber" and the "bombees" can accept it (with a sense of humor) as being a valuable learning experience and can proceed pronto with "Plan B." Successes are then more exciting to everyone involved.

The aforementioned are some of the necessary ingredients in facilitating learning taking place in the classroom. But there is yet another requisite — the BIG IDEA — humanness! Liberal amounts of acceptance, understanding, stroking, kindness, indulgence, humoring, flexibility, and accommodation need to be thrown into the pot in order for the pièce de résistance to be complete. "Building human relationships" — where have you heard that before?

Quite often it is difficult for teachers (established or otherwise) to understand the importance of humanness, especially if their style has been to "run a tight ship." They may view this technique as being so much more garbage to foul up the system. What they may not see is that "firmness with understanding" is very workable.

Try the BIG IDEA! You may discover that you like it.

introducing/ reinforcing the use of behavioral objectives

What are *you* doing to assist your students in LEARNING? in FEELING? in DOING?

You have already demonstrated that you are a "concerned professional" because

1. You have bought, borrowed, or stolen this book; and
2. You are reading it right now.

Whether or not you agree with all that is written here, there are some visible signs of growth you are exhibiting by merely examining the content herein. You are obviously

1. not one of those educators who is still naive enough to believe that the achievement of a degree has provided you with all of the knowledge, the methods, and the techniques that will ever be needed to achieve success in teaching;
2. convinced that education is neither dull, nor lifeless, nor unchanging;
3. not going to settle for being a "practicing incompetent"; and
4. aware of your responsibilities in providing your students with the opportunity to develop their latent capabilities.

HOORAY FOR YOU!!

21

Student Goals: Student Objectives

Think of yourself as an architect. Rather than designing a home to meet the needs of a family or a factory to meet the needs of an industrial company, you have the responsibility of designing learning experiences to meet the needs of your students. They are your clients. They embark on their education with excitement, with fear, with expectations, with joy. You become a very important person in the lives of your children. They place their trust in you to provide the experiences that they need to develop their abilities. They expect you to help them achieve the skills that they need to be successful in your class and to acquire the degree of proficiency necessary to cope successfully with the experiences that will be provided by their next teacher.

As the architect, it is important to study your clients. You need to know the general characteristics of growth and development for their age levels. Within this broad framework, you rapidly become aware of the individual differences in emotional, social, physical, and intellectual development. As you work with your class, you learn more about the present state of your students' skills in reading, writing, speaking, drawing, manipulating objects, and coping with daily problems.

All of this information becomes the baseline data to be used:

1. In selecting the concepts to teach toward that are of importance for your students;
2. In identifying the competencies in the general behavioral objectives that your students should be able to display;
3. In selecting the specific method that will be used to provide an opportunity for the students to develop the stated competency; and
4. In selecting the appropriate conditions within which the learning experience will occur.

In essence, you are an architect of living. You are focusing on the needs, interests, and capabilities of your students in planning and designing the classroom activities which they will experience. You have not fallen into the trap of focusing on content without consideration of the clients who are entrusted to you.

We would be highly critical of an architect who designed a nine-bedroom house for a family of three or who directed the builder to put up a shell for a person who had no skills to complete the structure.

Are we equally critical of what we do in the classroom? Think about it. Do you "dump" more factual information on your students than they have need of or interest in at this time? Do you provide classroom experiences that will ensure failure for a portion of the class because they do not possess the abilities to accomplish the tasks?

Before you respond with a quick "Of course I don't!" and feel insulted that these questions are being asked of a dedicated professional, how much do you REALLY know about your students? So often, even those of us who consider ourselves dedicated and student-oriented make assumptions about our students that would be found to be in error if we had factual information.

Elementary classroom teachers tend to have much more information available to them about their students than do secondary teachers. The elementary teachers not only have the permanent records of their students but also have hours of experiences with their students on an all-day, everyday basis. Even then, many teachers tend to consider this information as interesting but not of prime importance in designing learning experiences.

Think of your present class. What is the range in the reading levels? Are you designing experiences so that the youngsters on the lower level of the range can succeed and at the same time help them improve their skills? Are you providing experiences to challenge the youngsters at the upper end of the scale? Are you primarily designing for the middle-range group because they make up the majority of the class?

Youngsters start their school life with great eagerness and enthusiasm. They have personal goals and personal objectives. They expect to succeed. When they do achieve, the eagerness and enthusiasm tends to be retained. However, when the school experience results in failure and frustration, the youngster's eagerness is dampened and replaced with an attitude of "What's the use of trying? I can't do it."

The challenge for the teacher is to design experiences that will help youngsters increase their knowledge while improving their skills and developing the all-important positive self-image.

The Conceptual Model

Earlier in this chapter it was stated that information about your students became baseline data to be used in selecting the concepts that are important to them. As classroom teachers you may or may not be familiar with the School Health Education Study[1] (S.H.E. Study).

Rather than focusing on the content areas usually associated with health education, the S.H.E. Study proposed that the health curriculum be organized in the following ten concepts:

1. Growth and Development Influence and Are Influenced by the Structure and Functioning of the Individual.
2. Growing and Developing Follow a Predictable Sequence, Yet Are Unique for Each Individual.
3. Protection and Promotion of Health Are Individual, Community, and International Responsibilities.
4. The Potential for Hazards and Accidents Exists, Whatever the Environment.
5. There Are Reciprocal Relationships Involving Man, Disease, and Environment.
6. The Family Serves to Perpetuate Man and Fulfill Certain Health Needs.
7. Personal Health Practices Are Affected by a Complexity of Forces, Often Conflicting.
8. Utilization of Health Information, Products, and Services Is Guided by Values and Perceptions.
9. Use of Substances That Modify Mood and Behavior Arises from a Variety of Motivations.
10. Food Selection and Eating Patterns Are Determined by Physical, Social, Mental, Economic and Cultural Factors.

Because of the lack of emphasis on the mental–emotional aspect of health, we added an eleventh concept[2]

11. Emotional Health Is Influenced by Interpersonal Relationships and Enhanced by an Understanding of the Factors Affecting Behavior.

As can be seen, these concepts are broad statements which are applicable to all levels of learning. All content areas would fit into one or more of them. Each concept has physical, mental, and social dimensions, and the focus can be placed on the cognitive, affective, or psychomotor domains.

After selecting the concepts that are applicable to the students, the teacher needs to focus on the students. There then comes into play the need to identify the competencies or abilities that the

[1] School Health Education Study, *Health education: a conceptual approach to curriculum design.* St. Paul, Minnesota: 3M Education Press, 1967.

[2] Scott, G.D. & Carlo, M.W. *On becoming a health educator.* Dubuque, Iowa: Wm. C. Brown Co., Publishers, 1974, p. 31.

students should be able to exhibit in relation to the content included in the conceptual statement. This brings us to behavioral objectives.

BEHAVIORAL OBJECTIVES

Some educators dismiss behavioral objectives as being of little value and look on them as a passing fad. We strongly disagree with this stance for several reasons.

First, when the objective is properly stated, it forces us to focus on the student rather than on our own objectives.

Second, the objective designates an expected behavior which the student is able to exhibit. This behavior can be demonstrated, observed, or measured. Thus, we have a built-in evaluative system. When the objective is shared with the students, they know what they are to do and when they have been successful in accomplishing the stated behavior.

Third, it provides guidance in designing the learning experiences.

There are two types of behavioral objectives: (1) general behavioral objectives and (2) specific behavioral objectives. If you want to make sure that you are focusing on your students, it is necessary to learn how to write both types of objectives.

GENERAL BEHAVIORAL OBJECTIVES

After selecting a concept that is applicable to your students, you will need to consider:

1. What content within the concept is important to these students at their stage of growth and development?
2. What competencies or abilities should these students be able to achieve with this content?

Notice that, at this point, you are not considering any specific ways to achieve the competencies. You are only thinking in broad, general terms. Now, you need to have a model for a general behavioral objective. Here is one that we have found very useful in helping teachers learn to write in behavioral terms.

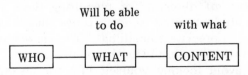

Let's apply the model by choosing one of the concepts and giving some examples of general behavioral objectives.

Concept 3:

Protection and promotion of health are individual, community, and international responsibilities.

General Behavioral Objectives:

1. The student will be able to identify ways to promote and protect the health of others.
2. The student will be able to describe the effects of littering on the health of the community.
3. The student will be able to explain ways that the health of others is dependent upon his/her own well-being.

As you can see, each of the examples fits the model:

WHO	will be able to do	WHAT	with what	CONTENT
1. The student	will be able to	IDENTIFY	ways to promote and protect the health of others	
2. The student	will be able to	DESCRIBE	the effects of littering on the health of the community	
3. The student	will be able to	EXPLAIN	ways that the health of others is dependent upon his/her own well-being	

These objectives are termed "general" because there is no one way designated to accomplish the behavior. There are many ways that could be chosen "to identify," "to describe," or "to explain." Likewise, there is no set focus in a stated dimension in the content. One could focus on the "physical" health, the "mental" health, or the "social" health of others or of the community.

One of the difficulties people have in writing objectives in behavioral terms is selecting verbs that designate behaviors rather than verbs that describe cognitive processes. Verbs such as "to recognize," "to understand," or "to appreciate" should be avoided. In each case, there is no way of observing or measuring these without asking, "What would students need to *do* to prove that they do recognize, understand, or appreciate something?" The answer to this question identifies the verbs that should have been used.

Likewise, avoid locking yourself into too specific a verb. The verb "to illustrate" is preferable to "to draw," "to color," "to cut," "to paint," or "to trace." Keep your options open until you are ready to write the specific behavioral objectives.

The following list may be of use to you.
Verbs to avoid in writing general behavioral objectives:

To know	To grasp the idea
To understand	To recognize
To appreciate	To become familiar with

Verbs to use in writing general behavioral objectives:

To demonstrate	To examine
To identify	To generate
To cite	To organize
To describe	To show
To explain	To prepare
To discuss	To assemble
To construct	To detect
To summarize	To analyze
To defend	To decide
To compile	To apply
To verify	To survey
To assess	To distinguish between
To select	To perform
To plot	To design
To illustrate	To plan
To discriminate between	To express
To compare	To create
To contrast	To make
To evaluate	To classify
To indicate	To develop

SPECIFIC BEHAVIORAL OBJECTIVES

You have a specific group of students for whom you will be planning. You know where their strengths and weaknesses lie. You know whether they need experiences to develop their eye–hand coordination, or their verbal, written, or reading skills. You know what interests they have and what their concerns are. In essence, you have a great deal of data about your students.

You now make use of these data in deciding which domain to focus on in writing the specific behavioral objective. If in your judgment the students need information, the focus selected would be in the cognitive domain. If the students already have factual information but need practice in applying these facts, then the focus selected would be in the affective domain. Placing the focus in the affective domain makes it possible for the students to express their interests in, their attitudes toward, their feelings about, or their emotions toward the information they have. On the other hand, perhaps the students need to develop their manipulative skills. In this case, the psychomotor domain would be the selected focus. In health education, the psychomotor domain is particularly useful in providing students with opportunities to express their ideas in visual ways, to organize their thoughts in writing, and to recall information by manipulating objects.

After selecting the domain, a choice of dimension is in order. You have three dimensions from which to choose — physical, mental-emotional, or social. The physical dimension refers either to how one is affected physically or to physical characteristics. In the mental-emotional dimension, the focus is either on the mind or the feelings. Recall, application, analysis, or evaluation are parts of the mental dimension. How one feels about something or as a result of some occurrence would be included in the emotional dimension.

An emphasis on the social dimension would refer to how others influence us, how we influence or affect others such as family members, friends, the community, and so forth.

As a general rule of thumb, only one domain and one dimension would be selected for any one learning experience. There are times, however, when it is very logical to use two or all three dimensions.

The selection of a domain and a dimension should be more than an empty exercise. Both must be reflected in the statement of the specific behavioral objective. If they aren't, then the chances that you will design the learning experience to emphasize these focal points are greatly reduced. A well-stated specific behavioral objective provides guidance in your designing efforts.

There are some criteria that should be applied to determine whether an objective is a specific behavioral objective:

1. It is *related* to the stated general behavioral objective. In other words, if the students successfully accomplish the specific behavior, they are on their way to attaining the general behavioral objective.

2. The *condition* under which the behavior will occur is clearly stated.

3. A specific behavior, ability, or action is given which can be *observed* or *measured.*

4. It is clearly stated *how* or in what form the behavior will occur.

5. The specific *content* from the concept is clearly stated.

Again, a model may be useful in helping you write specific behavioral objectives. The "blocks" do not have to be in the given order. All that is important is that each part of the model is represented in the objective.

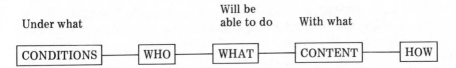

Look at the examples below:

Concept 2:

Emotional health is influenced by interpersonal relationships and enhanced by an understanding of the factors affecting behavior.

General Behavioral Objective:

The student will be able to cite the relationship between needs, feelings, and behavior.

Domain: Psychomotor   *Dimension:* Mental–Emotional

Specific Behavioral Objectives:

    1. After listening to the story of Freddy, the Friendly Bear Cub, the students will be able to portray the needs and feelings by acting out the story.

Domain: Affective   *Dimension:* Mental–Emotional

    2. Given a series of stem sentences, the student will be able to describe, in writing, the events that cause him/her to feel a specific emotion.

Domain: Cognitive   *Dimension:* Mental–Emotional

    3. Using the completed "Events Cause Feelings" worksheet, the student will be able to identify the emotion and the behavior or event in each sentence by listing them on an activity sheet.

Concept 4:

The potential for hazards and accidents exists, whatever the environment.

General Behavioral Objective:

The student will be able to identify ways of preventing physical injuries in a variety of environments.

Domain: Cognitive   *Dimension:* Physical

Specific Behavioral Objective:

4. Given a list of school environments from which to choose, the student will be able to describe two ways to prevent physical injury by making a poster with a slogan.

In each case, the specific behavioral objective meets the criteria and fits the model:

Under what | CONDITIONS |————————| WHO |

1. | After listening to the story . . . | | the student |

2. | Given a series of stem sentences . . . | | the student |

3. | Using the completed . . . worksheet | | the student |

4. | Given a list of school environments, | | the student |

will be able to do | WHAT |————— with what | CONTENT |

1. | will be able to portray | | the needs and feelings |

2. | will be able to describe | | the events that cause . . . emotion |

3. | will be able to identify | | the emotion and the behavior or event |

4. | will be able to describe | | ways to prevent physical injury |

| HOW |

1. | by acting out the story |

2. in writing

3. by listing them on an activity sheet

4. by making a poster with a slogan

People who haven't worked extensively with specific behavioral objectives tend to get confused over the focus on a domain. These questions are commonly raised:

1. "They have to use factual information, so why isn't it in the cognitive domain?"
2. "Writing is a skill. They're writing the answers, so why isn't it in the psychomotor domain?"

These are legitimate questions. The answers lie on where one is placing the emphasis. Look at the portions of two specific behavioral objectives.

1. . . . the student will be able to write a paragraph about one event that made him/her feel happy.
2. . . . the student will be able to describe, in writing, the events that cause him/her to feel specific emotions.

In the first example, the ability that is being focused on is the writing of a paragraph. In the second, the important behavior is the ability to describe the events. Here, the writing is only a means to attain an end.

The answer to the first question is somewhat similar. The knowledge the students have will be used in every learning experience. If the emphasis is on the attaining of facts, then the focus is on the cognitive domain. However, if the focus is on using the facts, then the ability being emphasized is either in the affective or the psychomotor domain.

The *key* to identifying the focus lies in the stated ability or the combination of the ability and the content. An example may clarify this point.

1. Given a list of eight people who influence their choice of health products, the students, individually, will be able to rank order them.

The stated ability is "to rank order." This objective is written with a psychomotor focus. Suppose, however, that the ability to write numbers from 1 to 8 isn't the important ability. A revision is in order.

1. Given a list of eight people, the students, individually, will be able to determine how much influence each has on their choice of health products by rank ordering.

Here the ability is "to determine the amount of influence each has." Since this ability involves personal opinion, the focus is on the affective domain. The rank ordering merely becomes the technique selected. Other techniques could have been chosen for the ⎡HOW.⎤

The suggestions that follow are not all-inclusive, but they may assist you in structuring specific behavioral objectives.

Suggestions for Conditions

After viewing the film	In class discussion
Given a series of . . .	After making a list
In small groups	While hearing a . . .
Individually	After listening to . . .
With a partner	As a homework assignment
Using the . . . worksheet	During an interview
Using a computer terminal	At learning stations

Suggestions for "How"

By values voting	By listing
By circling a picture	By interviewing . . .
By solving the . . . puzzle	By answering . . .
Verbally	By responding to . . .
In writing	By completing the stem sentences
By drawing pictures	By playing . . . game
By making a poster	By writing a spot announcement
By answering questions	By helping to . . .
By making a mobile	By making a collage
By placing . . . on a forced choice ladder	By matching
By drawing the correct pathway	By unscrambling the letters

With a little practice, you will find that objectives written in behavioral terms become very easy to construct. As you work with them, we think that you will see how they make you focus on your students and their needs. As you design the learning experiences directed by the objectives, you will, indeed, be assisting your youngsters in what education is all about — Learning, Feeling, and Doing.

designing learning experiences

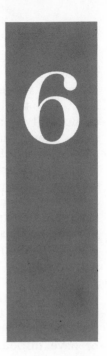

The elementary classroom teacher faces a special challenge of weaving together all portions of the educational program. There is a tendency to separate and compartmentalize the various content areas without utilizing multidisciplinary opportunities. Health education is one of the areas that permeates every aspect of living. Yet it is also one of the areas in which children tend to be short-changed. We would make a plea to elementary teachers not only to schedule time for health education sometime during the week but also to look for opportunities where content from the concepts could logically be a part of other subject areas.

Consider using learning experiences planned in the psychomotor domain for art lessons. Certain experiences in the Concepts (1 and 2) dealing with growth and development can logically be included as arithmetic lessons. Other experiences can be included in science, spelling, English, or social studies. The opportunities are there when one looks for them.

Planning Format

The designing of learning experiences is an ongoing responsibility. The role of the teacher can be compared with that of a restaurant chef. The chef must vary the menu, plan food combinations that appeal to the diner's palate, and plan the chef's "special." The restaurant will lose customers if the menu or the food is not acceptable. The teacher has a captive audience, thus the "customers" cannot opt for another "chef." Instead, where the teacher serves the same "menu" and makes no attempt to appeal to the learner's needs and interests, the students respond with a variety of behaviors. Students can lose their enthusiasm for learning, become bored, develop habits of truancy, and/or exhibit disruptive behavior patterns.

One of the most challenging responsibilities any teacher has is the designing of experiences which guide students through a sequential learning process. Designing takes both time and creativity, but the effort is very rewarding when youngsters respond with interest and enthusiasm.

There is no format that will be acceptable to everyone. Develop one that meets *your own* needs. While you are experimenting, we wish to suggest two which have proved to be useful to others.

Teachers who have a limited background in health information or have difficulty in matching the design with the stated specific behavioral objectives have found the first format extremely valuable. They state that having the objective written beside the design tends to keep them on the right track. Another advantage is having the content adjacent to the procedure.

Format 1

Concept:

General Behavioral Objective:

Domain: *Dimension:*

Introduction:

Specific Behavioral Objective	Procedure	Content	Teaching Aids
	Follow-up		

Some teachers have been working for years with objectives written in behavioral terms. Perhaps they couple this with an extensive knowledge of health information. Teachers who fall into this category find Format 2 to be the more useful.

Format 2

Concept:

General Behavioral Objective:

Domain: *Dimension:*

Specific Behavioral Objective:

Introduction:

Directions:

Learning Experience:

Follow-Up Procedure:

Utilizing either of these formats will help you to analyze your total teaching efforts. You will readily be able to observe if you are over-emphasizing any one domain of learning or any particular teaching/learning method. Adjustments can then be made to modify these overindulgences.

Designing for Student Involvement

Elementary teachers do a fantastic job of involving their young-sters in the classroom experiences. It is equally important in health education.

When you use the data about your students, when you write objectives in behavioral terms, when you design learning experiences to make it possible for the youngsters to exhibit the stated behaviors, then you can't avoid involving students in their own learning. When they own a piece of the action, they feel more responsible for the outcome.

Help your students to learn *because of you* rather than *in spite of you!*

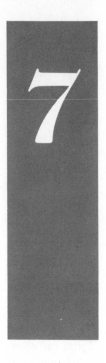

7 try these and then...

Systematic Planning

Experienced as well as neophyte facilitators of learning have, on the whole, demonstrated a propensity to be curious and receptive to education. Most recognize a very real need to recycle their own skills periodically so that they can, in turn, continue to make an impact on the people within their influence area. In this retooling process, teachers need a point of departure from which they can boldly plunge forward in the game of keeping up with changes in education. The old and familiar becomes a comfortable base upon which to build. Since all teachers in some form "plan" for the daily lessons, a logical departure base could be learning to redesign lessons with a different focus.

Many teachers have not given serious thought to lesson designing since their required collegiate experiences in the education department. It's not that they *don't* plan or predeliberate, but rather that the planning tends not to occur in a systematic way. The "planning" often is a mental process with only as much put in writing as is required by the school system for use by substitute teachers. There is rarely a systematic consideration of questions such as:

1. What have the students already experienced in prior grades?

Are the same things being dumped on them that they had last year, the year before, and the year before that? Some repetition is desirable, but there is a point at which it becomes nonproductive, dysfunctional, and turns kids off with a loud thud.

2. What domain of learning (cognitive, affective, psychomotor) within the present concept has received the major focus?

Has the only emphasis been placed on cognitive learning?

Students need to be more than walking storehouses of isolated facts. They need opportunities to draw on facts to express their ideas and opinions and to develop their manipulative skills. They need experiences that will help them develop their abilities to speak, to make decisions, to write, to draw, to construct, and so on. By developing these skills they are being provided with opportunities to make decisions — and making decisions is what education is all about.

3. What dimension of health (physical, emotional, social) within the present concept has received the major focus?

Learning to cope with emotional and social reactions is of vital importance. It is very common, however, for the emphasis to be placed only on the physical dimension. For example, how often does one focus only on the possibility of foods high in sugar content causing tooth decay or loss of teeth — without considering focusing on the feelings children have when they lose a tooth naturally or have to go to the dentist for a filling or an extraction? And how often does one focus on the social implications — the reactions of family and friends to the sight of obviously decayed teeth, to the missing tooth, or to the expressed apprehensions of the pending dental appointment?

Helping students develop their coping skills is an important goal in health education.

4. What individual differences are there in this class for which I need to design different learning experiences?

While some of the differences are obvious, other differences are easily hidden. The child for whom English is a second or third language is very apparent, as is the youngster who is deaf, blind, has a speech impediment, or whose reading ability is drastically below his peers. Less obvious is the student who has a visual problem that distorts words, one who has a slight loss of hearing, or one whose reading ability is only one or two levels below that of his classmates.

Teachers continually need to be aware of the importance of assisting students in coping with the normal learning frustrations

while the problems are still minor. Each time the student is successful it becomes a personal triumph. While it may not be as dramatic as
"Eureka!" or the proverbial light bulb going on, day-by-day accom-
plishments accumulate and the student's self-image improves. He can
achieve; he can accomplish; he can succeed! Success breeds success!
Contrarily, the student who suffers small frustrations day after day
reacts very normally. He gets discouraged. Continual lack of success
turns off the desire to try. Failure becomes predictable. His self-
image is that of a loser. The self-fulfilling prophecy has run full
circle. "I can't do it, so why should I try?"

Why all this discussion? To reemphasize to all teachers that they
must not write off *any* student. They must provide every possible
opportunity for learning for *every* youngster at every level. No one
will ever say that it is an easy task to help human beings develop,
but teachers can really underwrite education by being enthusiastic
and giving of themselves and their skills above and beyond the
routine. One of the keys to success is getting to know "the workers"
as well as "the work."

Experienced teachers will read this and say, "This is nothing
new. I've been doing this for years!" But have they really? It seems
to be relatively unusual when teachers of their own accord will plan
in writing. There seems to be a built-in ratio: the more teaching
experience under the belt, the fewer detailed written plans.

Designing and Redesigning

In workshop situations, teachers report that they feel little need
to write out plans because they have used a lesson several times and
"know it." — it has become part of their repertoire. Thus, they feel
very comfortable with the "tried and true." Where they are request-
ing assistance in their retooling effort is either in designing learning
experiences in the affective and psychomotor domains or in redesigning cognitive lessons into learning experiences that involve students
in the learning process.

This chapter is designed to respond to the desire of teachers
to *recycle* their skills and to the need for the professional *to develop*
the skill of designing. Hopefully, the examples given will provide the
impetus — much as a rocket gives the original thrust to a space ship —
for the professional to take off and fly on his/her own designing by:

1. Suggesting a format to use in designing;

2. Presenting a variety of learning experiences that have been used successfully in health education classes at the various skill levels in elementary schools;

3. Providing learning experiences for each of the eleven major concepts that encompass all of the content areas of health education.

Even though a specific format is utilized in all of the learning experiences, it is not implied that this representation is the *only* way. We suggest, however, that even the experienced teacher utilize some format and *write out* his or her plans until the inclusion of the following components of design becomes instinctive:

1. The major health concept being utilized;

2. The general behavioral objective that represents either the facet of the concept being pursued or the outcome of learning being sought;

3. The domain of learning reflecting the kind of learning that will take place in the experience;

4. The dimension of health being incorporated within the objective;

5. The specific behavioral objective(s) being chosen that will describe student behaviors to be performed and that will reflect the domain of learning and the dimension of health that will guide the learner to the accomplishment of the stated general behavioral objective;

6. Directions for the learner that will describe the steps to be taken to achieve the specific behavioral objective, and

7. Possible follow-ups that may serve to enrich the learning experience.

The reader will note that each of the sample learning experiences that follow is structured in this design. Try some of these and then . . . take off and fly with your own wings. You may be surprised at how amazingly strong these wings are — capable of carrying you to new heights. Soar, baby, soar!

concept 1:

Growth and Development Influence and Are Influenced by the Structure and Functioning of the Individual

Introduction to Concept — Lower Elementary Level[1]

DO THIS, DO THAT

Raise your hand if you have black or brown skin color!
Raise your hand if you have white skin color!
Raise your hand if you have a different colored skin!

Clap your hands if you have blue eyes!
Clap your hands if you have brown eyes!
Clap your hands if you have different colored eyes!

Stand up if you are a girl! Now sit.
Stand up if you are a boy! Now sit.

Raise your left hand if you are left handed!
Raise your right hand if you are right handed!

Shake your head if you look more like your mother than your dad!
Shake your head if you look more like your dad than your mom!
Shake your head if you resemble someone else in your family more than either of your parents!

Scratch your head if you have blonde hair!
Scratch your head if you have brown hair!
Scratch your head if you have reddish colored hair!
Scratch your head if you have black hair!

Tap your nose if you feel it is very long!
Tap your nose if you feel it is very short!

[1] Mary Elaine Seidenwand, School of Public Health, University of Michigan, Ann Arbor, Michigan.

If you feel you are very tall for your age, shake your hands!

If you feel you are short for your age, shake your hands!

If you feel your height is just about right for your age, shake your hands!

If you think you are good at drawing or making things with your hands, stand up and point to the sky! Now sit.

If you think you are not very good at drawing or making things with your hands, stand up and point to the ground! Now sit.

If you are a very fast runner, stand up and pretend you are running very swiftly! Now sit.

If you like to run but are not quite as fast as some of the other kids, stand up and pretend you are running rather slowly! Now sit.

If you don't like to run because you are very slow, just stand up! Now sit.

Why are some puppies born a different color from the mother dog?

Why do some people have a different skin color than others?

Why are some puppies born male and some female?

Why are some people born boys and some born girls?

Why are there different breeds of dogs?

Where do each and every one of us get all of these things that make us different from other people?

Our parents are responsible. When they mated (just as dogs or cats or other animals do), they passed their traits on to us. This is called HEREDITY.

A Gift To Me, My Heredity

Concept:

Growth and development influence and are influenced by the structure and functioning of the individual.

General Behavioral Objective:

The student will be able to identify characteristics which are influenced by heredity.

Domain: Cognitive   *Dimension:* Social

Grade Level: Lower elementary

Specific Behavioral Objective:

By completing a worksheet, the student will be able to identify the parents and/or grandparents who have characteristics similar to his/her own.

Directions: (Teacher)

1. Reproduce "A Gift To Me, My Heredity" (p. 43).
2. Reinforce explanation of "trait" and "heredity."
3. Read the statements to the class.

Directions: (Student)

1. Each statement describes something about you.
2. Which of your parents or grandparents is also like this (has this same trait)?
3. Color one block beside *each* person who has the same trait that you do.
4. Count the number of blocks that are colored in for each person.
5. Which one has the most colored blocks?

WHO AM I LIKE?

1. I am (right/left) handed like . . .
2. I have a nose like . . .
3. My eyes are the same color as . . .
4. My skin is the same color as . . .
5. I am (short/tall) like . . .
6. I have (straight/curly) hair like . . .

Suggested Follow-Up:

1. Discuss:
   a. others in the family who have similar traits — e.g., brothers, sisters, aunts, uncles.
   b. other traits that weren't mentioned — e.g., freckles.
2. Draw a family portrait in color. During "open house" have parents identify their family.

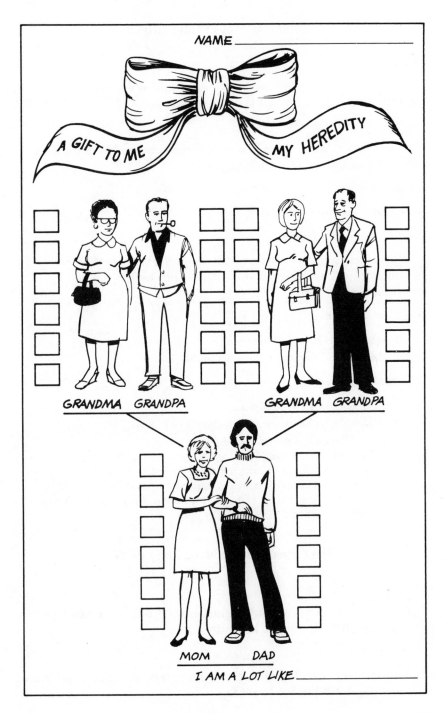

Wonderful Ways I Have Grown

Concept:

Growth and development influence and are influenced by the structure and functioning of the individual.

General Behavioral Objective:

The student will be able to demonstrate an understanding of the different dimensions of personal growth.

Domain: Cognitive   *Dimension:* All

Grade Level: Lower elementary

Specific Behavioral Objective:

By completing the "Wonderful Ways I Have Grown" checklist, the student will be able to show the ways he/she has grown in all dimensions since birth.

Directions: (Teacher)

1. Duplicate copies of "Wonderful Ways I Have Grown" (p. 45).
2. If necessary, read the statements to the class.

Suggested Follow-Up:

1. Read statements by sections.
2. Students raise hands for statements they checked.
3. Pause after each dimension to discuss:
   a. What other ways would you like to develop in this dimension?
   b. Of the items checked, which is most important to you?
   c. Of the items checked, which is least important to you?
   d. Why are some things important to some people and not very important to others?

The Case of the Growing Body Parts

Concept:

Growth and development influence and are influenced by the structure and functioning of the individual.

General Behavioral Objective:

The student will be able to demonstrate an understanding of growth being a continuing process.

44

Wonderful ways I have grown.

DIRECTIONS: PUT A CHECK (v) BY EACH SENTENCE WHICH DESCRIBES YOU.

PHYSICAL
SINCE BIRTH

____ 1. I HAVE GROWN TALLER.

____ 2. I HAVE GAINED WEIGHT.

____ 3. MY HAIR HAS GROWN LONGER.

____ 4. MY FEET HAVE GROWN.

MENTAL

____ 5. I HAVE LEARNED TO WRITE.

____ 6. I HAVE LEARNED MY A, B, C'S.

____ 7. I HAVE LEARNED TO READ.

____ 8. I HAVE LEARNED TO COUNT TO 100.

SOCIAL

____ 9. I SHARE MY THINGS WITH OTHER PEOPLE.

____ 10. I HELP MY FAMILY BY KEEPING MY ROOM CLEAN.

____ 11. I AM KIND TO OTHERS.

____ 12. I OBEY SCHOOL RULES.

EMOTIONAL

____ 13. I CRY WHEN I DON'T GET MY WAY.

____ 14. I AM HAPPY ONLY WHEN THE SUN IS SHINING.

____ 15. I'M NOT A POOR SPORT, EVEN WHEN I'M LOSING.

Domain: Cognitive   *Dimension:* Physical

Grade Level: Lower elementary

Specific Behavioral Objective:

In class discussion, the student will be able to identify verbally the various body parts that grow.

Directions:

1. Read Part I of the story "The Case of the Growing Body Parts" (p. 46).
2. Students compile list for Barney.
3. Read Part II (p. 48).

Suggested Follow-Up:

1. Construct a "Case of the Growing Body Parts" bulletin board.
2. Include a "Good Citizen" citation to the class from Barney Derby for the students' help in completing his mission.
3. Make "flash cards" of the body parts. Glue small pieces of magnetic tape on the back. Classify the parts by placing each in proper column: "Growth Seen" or "Growth Unseen."

THE CASE OF THE GROWING BODY PARTS

Part I

It seemed that Barney Derby had much more on his mind than usual today. The mission he was about to begin was one which he must complete quickly and carefully.

"Make NO mistakes!" the Chief had said. "The security and health of our entire nation — men, women, and children — is in *your* hands."

"Whew," Barney exclaimed as he drove away rapidly but carefully. The thought of having this much responsibility for the security and health of the whole nation was almost too much for his mind to handle. As if speaking to a passenger in the seat beside him, Barney declared aloud, "This must be *some case!*"

Before he knew it, Barney was at the place where he would be given the details of his mission. Barney's mind had been so caught in the tight web of a dream that he had scarcely noticed or enjoyed the beautiful countryside he loved. Barney shook his head and knew he must get down to business.

The deep silence was broken as Barney opened the car door and pushed away the gravel beneath his boot. His eyes carefully searched the surrounding area. No, no suspicious looking characters here, he thought to himself.

Slowly, he walked over to the phone booth, closed the door behind him, and began dialing the numbers that the Chief had given him— 0-0-7. "If I didn't know better, I'd think this was a movie," thought Barney.

A tape recording began to play, just as Barney had been told that it would. A cold, hard voice recited the instructions as Barney listened carefully.

"Get (*Teacher's name*)s (*Grade Level*) grade class to talk. They're the only ones who could give us the information our top scientists need to finish the Body Parts Project. The scientists still need the names of the body parts that grow.

"These students are the only ones who can provide us with a complete listing.

"Remember, this is super-secret information. Your mission, should you decide to accept it, is to get that list from the class—and, Barney, BE CAREFUL! . . . I've heard that those students can be pretty rough rascals! Good luck!!

"This tape will self-destruct in 5 seconds and the 0-0-7 phone number will no longer be in service."

Barney got back in his car and called Secret Operations on his radio phone.

"Give me (*Teacher's name*)'s address," he snapped. Then he put his car in gear and drove rapidly to the address he'd been given. As he drove by, he carefully looked to see if there was anyone around. To be on the safe side, he parked on the next street and casually strolled up to the house. After glancing around to see that he hadn't been followed, he pushed the doorbell. The door opened.

"Good evening, (*Teacher's name*). I'm Barney Derby and here's my identification. Your country needs the help of you and your class. May I come in?"

"Of course, do come in and tell me what we can do to help."

End of Part I

To Students:

1. Since the health and security of our great nation depends on whether or not we share our knowledge, should we make a list for Barney?
2. He needs a list of the parts of the body that grow. Remember, though, there may be a spy among us that will try to put a wrong answer on the list.
3. Let's not forget that there are parts inside of our bodies we can't see that grow too.
4. Let's make two separate lists. One list of the body parts we can see; another list of the body parts we can't see.
5. Are there any other body parts we should include on our list before handing it over to Barney?

Part II

After leaving (*Teacher's name*)'s house, Barney quickly turned up the collar of his old grey rain coat, pulled his black hat over one eye, and walked rapidly to his car.

Not daring even to glance at the words written on the paper, Barney stuffed the lists into a plain brown envelope.

He drove without stopping for what seemed like hours. Finally, by nightfall he arrived at the place where he was to make his delivery. Inside a large grey building several top scientists were pacing the floor frantically and wondering if Barney would ever arrive.

When they saw the flash of his headlights, they were very happy. It seemed like ages until Barney walked through the secret passageway.

"Thank you, thank you," the scientists kept repeating as Barney handed them the small brown envelope.

Barney, barely hearing what they were saying, suddenly felt very weary. It seemed as if the weight of the world had been lifted from his shoulders. For the first time that day, he noticed that his stomach was empty, growling for food. His mouth was very dry.

"How ever did you do it?" Barney heard the scientists ask.

All that Barney could do was bow his head and reply, "Oh, it's all in a day's work, but the real credit goes to (*Teacher's name*) (*Grade Level*) grade class.

concept 1:

Growth and Development Influence and Are
Influenced by the Structure and Functioning
of the Individual

Introduction to Concept — Upper Elementary Level

NOT FOR SALE — ME!

How familiar does this sound to you? "You're too *old* for that!"
Or how about this? "Why, I thought you'd grown out of that state!"
I'll bet these are expressions that you're almost as used to hearing as
your very own name. Yes, you may have grown too old for diapers,
too big for that favorite T-shirt, or too smart for someone to cheat
you at a game of Monopoly. But did you realize there is something
you will never be too old, too big, or too smart for? That's for
growing and developing.

Each part of your body, from the tiniest cell to the largest body
system, is constantly growing or developing and will continue to do
so throughout your entire lifetime. Even when you celebrate your
12th, 24th, 48th, or 96th birthday, parts of your body still will be
either growing or developing.

Whether you've noticed it or not, you do have some say in the way
your body grows and develops. Your actions, as well as your feelings,
can help you or hurt you.

To Students:

1. What are some things you do that help your growth?
2. What are some things you do that hinder (hurts) your growth?
3. What are some things you do that help your development?
4. What are some things you do that hurt your development?

Notice that these are all things you can change if you really want to.
You do have a strong influence on the way your body grows, de-

velops, or changes. But the very structure of your body also plays an important role in this process.

Unlike those things we talked about earlier, these are some things we cannot change at will. Our heart continues to pump blood, our skeleton offers support and protects our internal organs, and built-in regulators signal our need for food or water, whether we give our consent or not.

We have no say, either, in such things as the color of our eyes, our hair, or our skin, the shape of our face; the size of our feet; whether we are boys or girls; how tall we will be. All of these things, which are called physical characteristics, we inherited. They are among the many traits or characteristics of our parents or grandparents that are passed on to us. This process of inheriting our physical traits and characteristics is called HEREDITY.

To Students:

> 1. Name some characteristics that are inherited which begin with
> the letters of the word "Heredity."

Sample:

H air color

E ye color

R ight- or left-handedness

E ars large or small

D imples

I ntelligence

T all or short

Y ellow, black, red, or white skin

Although at times we might wish we could change some of these traits, they are like items we buy on sale — NONRETURNABLE. However, in one sense, they are RECYCLABLE. They are traits which we may, in turn, pass on to our own children.

To Students:

> 1. What are some of your characteristics that you would want to
> pass on to your children?

In this concept we will be LEARNING about our heredity and about the parts of our body and how they function. We will be looking at our FEELINGS about our own characteristics and ways we have grown emotionally. Finally, we will take a look at what we are DOING or could be doing to improve our health and promote our own growth and development.

Inherited or Acquired?

Concept:

Growth and development influence and are influenced by the structure and functioning of the individual.

General Behavioral Objective:

The student will be able to identify inherited and acquired characteristics.

Domain: Cognitive   *Dimension:* Mental

Grade Level: Upper elementary

Specific Behavioral Objective:

After making a list of personal characteristics, the student will be able to differentiate between acquired and inherited characteristics by labeling a partner's list.

Directions: (Student)

1. Make a list of your own traits or characteristics.
2. Include not only the obvious physical characteristics, but also those that are emotional, social, or mental.
3. Choose a partner and exchange lists.
4. On your partner's list:
   a. Put an "I" if the trait is inherited.
   b. Put an "A" if the trait is acquired.

Suggested Follow-Up:

Discussion:
1. Review lists as identified.
2. What is one characteristic that other members of your family inherited, but you did not?

3. What are some of the traits or characteristics that you would like to acquire?
4. How might you try to develop these?

Body Defenses Word Scramble

Concept:

Growth and development influence and are influenced by the structure and functioning of the individual.

General Behavioral Objective:

The student will be able to cite protective mechanisms of the body.

Domain: Cognitive   *Dimension:* Mental

Grade Level: Upper elementary

Specific Behavioral Objective:

In dyads, the student will be able to identify protective mechanisms of the human body by solving a word scramble puzzle.

Directions: (Teacher)

1. Reproduce copies of the "Word Scramble" (p. 53).
2. Organize the class in dyads.
3. Key for "Word Scramble":

1. Tears	7. White blood cells
2. Blood	8. Nails
3. Eyelids	9. Spinal fluid
4. Body Temperature	10. Bones
5. Eyelashes	11. Lymph nodes
6. Skin	12. Outer ear

Suggested Follow-Up:

1. Classify each defense mechanism by body system.
2. List the specific protective devices of various animals — e.g.,
   Porcupines — quills
   Skunk — ejection of offensive smelling musky liquid
   Bees — stingers
   Bears — claws, heavy fur
   Toads/Frogs — protective coloration

WORD SCRAMBLE

Directions:

Mr. Peabody spent several hours after school one day putting up a bulletin board about protective devices of the human body. When he came to class the following morning, however, he found all the letters had fallen off of the board. His class lesson on body defenses is scheduled for today. Unscramble the letters so that Mr. Peabody can still use the board to help present his lesson. Some of the letters are already in place.

1. RASTE   _ _ A _ _
2. DLOOB   _ _ _ O _
3. DEILEYS   _ Y _ L _ _ _
4. ODBY   PETEUERMATR
      _ _ D _   _ E _ _ E R _ T _ _ _
5. LEHSSYEAE   E _ _ _ _ S _ E _
6. NISK   _ _ I _
7. HETIW   DLOOB   SCLEL
      _ _ _ T _   _ _ _ _ D _ _ E _ _ _
8. SLAIN   _ A _ _ _
9. NIALPS   DILUF   S _ _ _ A _   _ _ U _ _
10. NESOB   B _ _ _ _
11. PYMLH   ONSED   _ _ _ _ H _ O _ _ _
12. TOERU   REA   _ U T _ _ _ A _

Handicapped: Are You or Am I?

Concept:

     Growth and development influence and are influenced by the structure and functioning of the individual.

General Behavioral Objective:

     The student will be able to give a personal opinion about people with handicaps.

Domain: Affective   *Dimension:* Emotional

Grade Level: Upper elementary

Specific Behavioral Objective:

While hearing a series of statements, the student will be able to indicate his/her feelings toward handicapped persons by values voting.

Directions: (Teacher)

1. Prepare four 5 X 8 cards labeled: "Strongly Agree," "Agree," "Disagree," "Strongly Disagree."
2. Laminating the cards will protect them for long-term usage.
3. Place the cards in different areas of the floor.

Directions: (Students)

1. As each statement is read, move to the position on the floor which expresses your personal opinion about the statement.

2. There is no "correct" response.

Statements: (Option 1)

1. I feel awkward when I'm around a person who is blind.
2. I feel uncomfortable talking to a person who wears a leg brace.
3. I would like to help a blind student with class assignments by being a "reader."
4. I would like to be a volunteer helper for the "Special Olympics."
5. I would be pleased to have a handicapped person as a friend.
6. I get angry when someone teases kids who have problems with learning or understanding.

Specific Behavioral Objective:

While hearing a series of statements, the student is able to predict his/her behavior when involved with handicapped people by values voting.

Statements: (Option 2)

1. If a boy in our class wore glasses, I would tease him.
2. If a girl in our class were blind, I would ask the teacher if I could help her with the class assignments.

3. If a boy in our class was hard of hearing, I would not talk to him.
4. When I see a person who walks with crutches, I stare at him/her.
5. If a boy in my class wore leg braces, I would choose him to be on my team (at recess/in physical education class).

Specific Behavioral Objective:

While hearing a series of statements, the student will be able to express an opinion about handicapped persons by values voting.

Statements: (Option 3)

1. People with handicaps should be given a chance to prove what they can do.
2. Every store should be required to provide a ramp so that people in wheelchairs can shop there as easily as the rest of us.
3. All schools should provide restroom stalls wide enough for people in wheelchairs.
4. There are so few people in wheelchairs that it would be a waste of money to require schools to put a drinking fountain low enough for them to use.
5. It's not fair to give handicapped people reserved parking spaces.
6. We are all handicapped in some way.

Suggested Follow-Up:

1. Discuss:
   a. why we may feel uncomfortable
   b. ways to overcome uncomfortable feelings
   c. how students would feel if they had that particular handicap
   d. how students would want to be treated if they were either temporarily or permanently handicapped
   e. how they can help handicapped students in the school

concept 2:

Growing and Developing Follow a Predictable
Sequence Yet Are Unique for Each Individual

Introduction to Concept — Lower Elementary Level[2]

MOTHER'S FAMILY ALBUM

It was a gloomy, rainy day. Johnny was tired of playing with his toys. He turned on the TV to watch his favorite program, but he'd seen it before. Johnny kept switching channels hoping to find a new show or a new cartoon.

"Johnny," his mother called from the kitchen, "you're going to break that television if you keep it up."

"Ah, Mom," whined Johnny, "I can't help it. I've seen all of the programs and I'm looking for a new one. There's nothing to do around here."

"Why don't you read one of your books or play with your toys?" inquired his mother.

"I'm tired of them. Mom, what else can I do?"

To Students:

What do you do on a rainy day?

"Well, let's see, now," said Mother as she entered the living room." Her eyes scanned the room in search of something to do.

"Nothing on the coffee table," she thought. Then her eyes stopped on a tattered binding of a book on the top shelf of the bookcase.

"Would you like to look at my family's photo album, Johnny?" asked his mother.

Johnny had never seen the old album before and his eyes lit up at the very thought of it.

[2] Developed by Dawn Hilston, Kent State University, Kent, Ohio

"Gee, Mom, that sounds like fun!" exclaimed Johnny.

Johnny's mother pulled the album off the shelf and gave it to him. He sat down on the floor, eagerly opened the album, and started to look at the photos. Johnny looked and looked first on one page and then on another, but he didn't recognize anyone.

"Mom, are you sure that this is *our* family album?" asked Johnny.

Johnny's mother laughed and said, "Yes, I'm sure it's our family album, but it's only one of them. These are pictures of my side of the family. Do you see the big brown and gold book on the top shelf? That's the family album on your dad's side of the family."

"Oh," said Johnny, "but I don't recognize anyone at all. Who are all of these people?"

"Let me see if I can help you out," said mother. "Bring it over and sit on the couch beside me."

"Who's the baby?" inquired Johnny as he pointed to a picture.

"Why, that's me, Johnny," she exclaimed.

"Is that really you Mom? Gee, you were such a little baby," said Johnny.

"Well, I was only six months old when that picture was taken, Johnny, and I've grown a lot since then."

"Who's this, Mom?" asked Johnny pointing to a young man standing next to a house.

"That's Grandpa Smith, Johnny," said mother.

"Aw, that can't be Grandpa. Grandpa Smith has white hair," said Johnny.

"Oh, Johnny," his mother laughed, "your Grandpa didn't always have white hair. When he was a young man, his hair was bright red. It was just like your Uncle Bob's is now."

To Students:

What color is your grandpa's hair? Was it always that color? Is anyone's grandpa bald? Was he always bald?

"Is this you, Mom?" asked Johnny pointing to another photo.

"Yes, I was about five year's old in that picture," said Mother.

"What are those things on your knees, Mom?" asked Johnny.

"Those are bandages. I was just learning to ride a two-wheeler and I wasn't very good at it yet," explained Mother.

"Who's the little boy in the picture with you?" asked Johnny.

"That's my cousin, Jeff. He was six months younger than I but, boy, could he ride a bike! He hardly ever fell off. I could swim better than he could, though. Let's see, I think there's a picture of us swimming in Grandpa's pond. Yes, here it is," said Mother.

To Students:

What skills did you have when you were 5 years old? What skills did you need help with? What skills were you looking forward to learning?

"Do you have some pictures of you in school, Mom?" asked Johnny.

"Oh, my yes!" exclaimed Mother. "Here's one of the first ones when I was in the first grade. That's Uncle Bob with me. He was in the third grade."

"What happened to your two front teeth? You sure look funny," laughed Johnny.

"Oh, I lost them somehow. I can't even remember how it happened, now," said Mother.

"My front teeth came out when I was in kindergarten," said Johnny. "What took you so long, Mom?"

"Each person grows at his own rate, Johnny, and the primary teeth come out when the permanent tooth that is growing below it pushes on it and loosens it. Mine came out when I was in the first grade and yours came out when you were in kindergarten. That was when it was time for us," exclaimed Mother.

To Students:

When did you lose your first tooth?

To Teacher:

Emphasize the range in ages.

"Where are Uncle Bob, Uncle Nick, and Aunt Sue?" inquired Johnny.

"Here's a picture of the whole family, Johnny. Can you figure out who's who?" asked Mother.

"There's Grandma and Grandpa Smith and Uncle Bob. Here you are. This must be Uncle Nick and that has to be Aunt Sue. Why is Aunt Sue taller than Uncle Nick? He's older than she is, isn't he?" asked Johnny.

"Yes," laughed Mother. "Aunt Sue is a year younger than Uncle Nick. When that picture was taken she was much taller than he was. It was a couple of years before Uncle Nick caught up with Aunt Sue. Now, he's over six feet tall. You know, Johnny, girls often grow faster than boys do. Boys start later but they keep growing after the girls stop. Of course, a lot depends on how tall your parents are," explained Mother.

"How tall will I be?" asked Johnny.

"I can't tell you that, Johnny. I guess we'll just have to wait and see. Look at this family picture again. Grandma Smith is 5 feet 3 inches tall and Grandpa is 5 feet 11 inches tall. Uncle Nick is taller than both of them. Aunt Sue is almost as tall as Grandpa. I'm 5 feet 7 inches tall and Uncle Bob is an inch shorter than I am. So, you see, in my family we are all taller than at least one of our parents, but there was no way of telling how tall any of us were going to be," explained Mother.

"O.K., but I hope I'm not as tall as Dad is," laughed Johnny.

"Well, then I hope you get your wish," laughed Mother, "but don't be disappointed if you take after your Dad's side of the family."

Their laughter was interrupted by the sound of a car pulling up in the driveway.

"Dad's home!" shouted Johnny as he ran to the door.

"Hey, Dad, come and see these funny pictures of Mom," Johnny yelled as he ran out of the house to meet his father.

To Students:

Have you ever wondered about growing up? What questions do you have?

Growing, Changing, And Rearranging

Concept:

Growing and developing follow a predictable sequence yet are unique for each individual.

General Behavioral Objective:

The student will be able to demonstrate an understanding that people grow and develop at different rates.

Domain: Affective   *Dimension:* Physical

Grade Level: Lower elementary

Specific Behavioral Objective:

After listening to a poem, the student will be able to evaluate his/her own growth and development by answering questions.

Directions: (Teacher)

1. Make up a poem on growth and development, or use the following example:

GROWING, CHANGING, AND REARRANGING

Were you once fat? Were you once small?
Are you now skinny? Are you now tall?
Has your hair grown? Has it become curly or straight?
Have you lost a tooth of recent or late?
Do your nails need cutting every week or so?
Does your mother exclaim, "My, how your feet do grow!"
Are your arms longer than your sleeves?
Are your pants rapidly approaching your knees?
If you can answer yes to a question or two,
You're on the way to learning something about you.
You're learning that you're growing in leaps and bounds,
You're finding that you're growing both up and around.
Some of you are growing at a very fast rate,
While the rest of you will have to wait.
But don't worry or frown, don't fret or stew,
Because when you're done growing, you'll be a unique you.

—Dawn Hilston

2. As students listen to the poem, have them think about how they are growing and developing.
3. Read the poem.
4. Repeat the questions from the poem and have the students verbally answer.

Suggested Follow-Up:

1. Write a poem:
    a. describing their own growth and development
    b. describing one thing about themselves that is unique
2. Draw two pictures with captions:
    a. how they look now
    b. how they looked two or three years ago

I'm Good At This — You're Good At That!

Concept:

Growing and developing follow a predictable sequence yet are unique for each individual.

General Behavioral Objective:

The student will be able to demonstrate an understanding of people growing and developing at different rates.

Domain: Cognitive   *Dimension:* Physical

Grade Level: Lower elementary

Specific Behavioral Objective:

After singing a song, the students will be able to cite examples of physical skills they have or don't have by participating in a discussion.

Directions: (Teacher)

1. Lecturette covering the following:
    a. How we grow and develop as we get older.
    b. As we grow and develop, we can do things that we couldn't before.
    c. We each have our own rate of development.
    d. This is one thing that makes us each a very special person.
    e. No two people are exactly alike. We are unique.

2. Select a song that has lyrics to act out:
   a. Teach motions for the song.
   b. Keep a tally on chalkboard of number of times song is sung.
   c. Students drop out when they can't keep up and note the number on board at that point.
   d. Sing the song with motions while increasing the speed each time.
3. Draw a continuum on chalkboard for tallies.
4. Note the number of students who dropped out at each interval.
5. Discussion:
   a. Our skill levels are different even though we are the same age.
   b. Some people are very good at singing songs very fast while doing motions, while others are very good at other things.
6. Put two columns on chalkboard, newsprint, or a clear acetate.
   a. Develop a list of physical skills they "Do very well" and "Don't do very well."
   b. Verbally compare the lists emphasizing a positive approach.

Suggested Follow-Up:

1. Discuss people who can do a skill well helping those who can't but want to be more skilled.

Height/Weight: Same or Different?

Concept:

Growing and developing follow a predictable sequence yet are unique for each individual.

General Behavioral Objective:

The student will be able to demonstrate an understanding of people growing and developing at different rates.

Domain: Cognitive   *Dimension:* Physical

Grade Level: Lower elementary

Specific Behavioral Objective:

In small groups the student will be able to compare the physical growth of three people by recording height and weight.

Directions: (Teacher)

1. Have student compute own age in years and months — e g., 7 years, 4 months.

2. Set up height and weight stations.

3. Form line from youngest to oldest.

4. Form small groups of students of same age (years and months).

5. Assign each group to a station.

6. Have each student record own height/weight and that of two other group members on the "Same or Different" worksheet, p. 63.

7. Have student compare the heights and weights of the three people and list in the proper column.

Suggested Follow-Up:

1. Discussion:

   a. How many had someone in your group of three who weighed the same as someone else? Who were the same height?

   b. How many had no one in your group who weighed the same? How many had no one who was the same height?

   c. You are the same age. Why aren't you the same height? Weight?

SAME OR DIFFERENT

My name: _____

My age: _____ years   _____ months

My height: _____ centimeters

My weight: _____ kilos

Fill in for two other members of your group.

Name: _____

Age: _____ years   _____ months

Height: _____ centimeters

Weight: _____ kilos

Name: _____

Age: _____ years   _____ months

Height: _____ centimeters

Weight: _____ kilos

Same Height or Weight	Different Height or Weight

Would You Rather . . . ?[3]

Concept:

Growing and developing follow a predictable sequence yet are unique for each individual.

General Behavioral Objective:

The student is able to demonstrate the differences in social development.

Domain: Affective   *Dimension:* Social

Grade Level: Lower elementary

[3] Developed by Janelle Falcone, Tallmadge (Ohio) Public Schools.

Specific Behavioral Objective:

Through values voting, the student will be able to indicate a personal preference when given a series of paired statements that involve social situations.

Introduction:

In the activity we are going to do there is no right or wrong choice. Sometimes we like to be alone. Sometimes we like to be with other people. Sometimes we would rather be with some people instead of other people. Any choice you make is O.K. Think about each statement. Which choice would you make most of the time? This is called "Would You Rather . . .?"

Directions:

1. Designate two corners of the room to be used for answers.
2. Have students *move* to the corner of their choice for each pair of statements. (All statements do not need to be used in the same session.)

Would You Rather:

— Play with just one friend?
— Play with a group of children?

— Play at home with my brothers, sisters, or friends?
— Play at home by myself?

— Talk to my mom or dad?
— Talk to my teacher?

— Eat at home with my family?
— Eat at school with my friends?

— Go someplace with my family?
— Go someplace with my friends?

— Do a job around the house by myself?
— Have my mom or dad help me with my job?

Suggested Follow-Up:

Discuss:

1. When would you rather be alone?
2. When would you rather be with one friend?
3. When would you rather be with a group of children?
4. When would you rather be with your parents?

It's Nice to Have a Friend[4]

Concept:

Growing and developing follow a predictable sequence yet are unique for each individual.

General Behavioral Objective:

The student is able to identify the factors that influence the development of social relationships.

Domain: Affective   *Dimension:* Social

Grade Level: Lower elementary

Specific Behavioral Objective:

When given a series of statements, the student is able to identify the behaviors that are important in a friend by rank ordering.

Directions:

It's nice to have a friend. What is more important to you in a friend? Rank in order the five items from "1" to "5" by putting a "1" in front of the thing that is *most* important, a "2" in front of the next most important, a "3," "4," and then a "5" in front of the thing that is *least* important to you.

A. __ Shares food, candy, or toys with me.

B. __ Keeps secrets I tell her/him.

C. __ Helps me when I am in trouble.

D. __ Tells me when I'm wrong.

E. __ Listens to what I have to say.

Suggested Follow-Up:

1. Draw a chart on chalkboard or a transparency (clear acetate).
   a. Tabulate the rankings for each phrase.
   b. Underline the highest number of tallies received by each phrase.
2. Which behavior is the *most* important to most of the people in the class?
3. If it wasn't the most important to you, why is your choice more important?
4. Which behavior is the *least* important to most of the people in the class?

[4] Developed by Cheryl Holloway, Tallmadge (Ohio) Public Schools.

Statement	1	2	3	4	5
A					
B					
C					
D					
E					

5. If you don't agree, why is one of the other behaviors less important to you?
6. What do you do for your friends?
7. What is a "friend"?
8. Which of your needs does a friend help you fill?

Sorry, We Can't Be Friends[5]

Concept:

Growing and developing follow a predictable sequence yet are unique for each individual.

General Behavioral Objective:

The student is able to identify the factors that influence the development of social relationships.

Domain: Affective   *Dimension:* Social

Grade Level: Lower elementary

Specific Behavioral Objective:

When given a series of statements, the student is able by rank ordering to identify the behaviors that keep friendships from developing.

[5] Developed by Cheryl Holloway, Tallmadge, (Ohio) Public Schools.

Directions:

Sometimes people do things to us that we don't like. Sometimes we do things to others that they don't like. If this happens often we won't be friends. What is the *worst* thing that a person could do to you? Rank the five behaviors from "1" to "5" with number "1" being the *worst*.

A. __ Tells others a secret I told her/him.

B. __ Tries to boss me.

C. __ Makes fun of me.

D. __ Tells lies about me.

E. __ Does not share food, candy, or toys with me.

Suggested Follow-Up:

1. Tally the items that were ranked "1" or "2."

2. Why do you think these behaviors are worse than the others that were listed?

3. Why would you not choose to be friends with people that act this way?

---

concept 2:

Growing and Developing Follow a Predictable Sequence Yet Are Unique for Each Individual.

Introduction to Concept — Upper Elementary Level

I AM DIFFERENT

Note to teacher:

To prepare for this introduction you will need to have available some of the following:

1. A record player

2. Musical records (without lyrics) of:

   a. a stirring march

   b. a classical selection

    c. pop music

    d. contemporary music

  3. An abstract drawing or painting in which the figures are undefined, or a transparency showing an optical illusion (overhead projector).

  4. A small box, with perforated holes in the lid, containing an object or objects with a distinct odor (slice of lemon, pine needles, spice, etc.).

  5. A box with an opening large enough for a student's hand to reach in and feel an object without the object being seen (suggested objects — a piece of fur, a nail, a sipping straw, a piece of popped popcorn, etc.).

Please put your head down on your desk and listen carefully. You are going to hear different kinds of music. Use your imagination and after each, tell us what you picture in your mind when you hear that music. (Repeat this procedure with each of the musical selections.)

Teacher:

    Hold up picture.

Look at this picture. If you were the artist what title might you give it? Please write your title on a piece of scratch paper. When everyone finishes, you may share your title with the class.

Here are two interesting boxes. One is a "smell" box and the other is a "touch" box. Pass each box around the room. When you get the "smell" box, do just that and write on your paper what comes to your mind when you smell that odor. *I don't want you to guess what the object in the box is.* Only write down what you picture in your mind. With the "touch" box, put your hand in and feel the object, and write down what you picture in your mind.

Will you share your thoughts with the class?

Did you enjoy doing these activities and using your imagination? I didn't ask you to do these things only to have fun, however. You heard all of the different thoughts that your classmates had. Can you tell us why we had so many different answers? Can you guess what my *big idea* was in having you do this activity?

Teacher:

    (It is hoped that the *big idea* was to demonstrate that everyone is different and everyone interprets things from a different point of view.)

Even though you are like other people in many ways, each of you is different from every other person in the world. There is no one else exactly like you. This is because of your heredity (the traits you receive from your parents) and all of the different experiences in living you have as you grow and develop. The more you learn and the more experiences you have, the more you grow physically, mentally, emotionally, and socially. This growing and developing goes on all of your life and makes you different from everyone else.

I AM DIFFERENT

I am different, don't you see?
Because you are you, and I am me.

When Did You First . . .?

Concept:

Growing and developing follow a predictable sequence yet are unique for each individual.

General Behavioral Objective:

The student will be able to demonstrate an understanding of people growing and developing at different rates.

Domain: Psychomotor   *Dimension:* Physical

Grade Level: Upper elementary

Specific Behavioral Objective:

As a homework assignment, the student will be able to chart his/her own physical growth and development by completing the "When Did You First . . .?" worksheet.

Directions: (Teacher)

1. Give each student a copy of the "When Did You First . . .?" worksheet (p. 71).
2. Have students take worksheet home. Have parents help.

Suggested Follow-Up:

1. Compare ages at which each skill was performed.
2. Make a continuum on the chalkboard of the range of ages on selected skills.
3. Discuss: "What evidence is there that people develop at different rates"?
4. Write a paragraph about "One Skill I'd Like to Develop This Year."
5. Discuss the paragraph in dyads.

Name: _____

WHEN <u>DID</u> YOU FIRST . . . ?

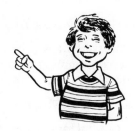

Directions: Write in the age at which you first performed the skill listed below. If you aren't sure on an item, ask your parents.

Skill	Approximate Age
1. Roll over	
2. Sit up alone	
3. Crawl	
4. Stand up alone	
5. Talk	
6. Walk	
7. Drink from a cup	
8. Feed yourself	
9. Run without falling	
10. Ride a tricycle	
11. Skip	
12. Do a forward roll	
13. Color in the lines	
14. Catch a ball	
15. Ride a bicycle without training wheels	
16. Print your own name	
17. Tie your shoes	
18. Wash your own hair	
19. Dress yourself without help	
20. Count to 100	
21. Learn alphabet	
22. Make your own bed	
23. Cross street by oneself	
24. Write your own name	
25. Help with chores around the house	

Recipe for Growing

Concept:

Growing and developing follow a predictable sequence yet are unique for each individual.

General Behavior Objective:

The student will be able to demonstrate an understanding of the relationship among heredity, experience, personal habits, and growth and development.

Domain: Affective   *Dimension:* All

Grade Level: Upper elementary

Specific Behavioral Objective:

Individually, the student will be able to identify the factors that contribute to personal growth and development by completing a recipe card.

Directions: (Teacher)

1. Provide a 3 X 5 card for each student.
2. Draw a large card on the chalkboard as per the example on p. 73. Use the headings only.
3. Have students put headings on own card.
4. What's Cooking? — MY RECIPE FOR GROWING
   a. List under "ingredients" all the physical, social, mental, and emotional factors you think are important to your own growth and development.
   b. Give directions.

Suggested Follow-Up:

1. Individually, read recipe aloud.
2. Discuss the ingredients stressing individual differences.
3. Display recipes on a Bulletin Board inside an outline of a cookbook (see p. 73).

Station K.N.O.W. — On the Go!

Concept:

Growing and developing follow a predictable sequence, yet are unique for each individual.

WHAT'S COOKING? _My Recipe For Growing_

FROM THE KITCHEN OF: _(Susie Jones)_

SERIES: _(1)_

INGREDIENTS: _(Good Food, Sunshine, Friends, Loving Family, Exercise, Rest, Heredity.)_

DIRECTIONS: _Mix together the above ingredients. Watch carefully._

BULLETIN BOARD IDEA

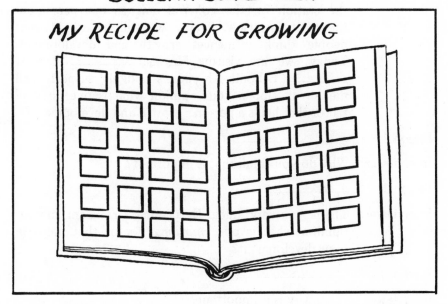

MY RECIPE FOR GROWING

The student will be able to demonstrate an understanding of the relationship among heredity, experience, personal habits, and growth and development.

Domain: Affective   *Dimension:* All

Grade Level: Upper elementary

Specific Behavioral Objective:

During a simulated person-on-the-street interview, the student will be able to explain factors that contribute to an individual's growth and development by discussing these factors.

Directions: (Teacher)

1. Use a microphone from a tape recorder or make one out of cardboard.
2. Interview students at random:

STATION K.N.O.W. — ON THE GO!

Interviewer: Hello, folks. I'm _____ from Station K.N.O.W. — the station on the go! Welcome to our person-on-the-street interview. Today we will be asking what people think influences growth and development; Today, we are visiting Mr./Ms. _____ class at _____ School. Ah, here's a likely suspect. Tell me, sir/ma'am, in your opinion what is one *physical* factor that helps a person's growth and development?

Person 1: _____

Interviewer: Why do you think that is important?

Person 1: _____

Interviewer: Thank you very much. Excuse me, sir/ma'am, in your opinion what is one *emotional* factor that helps in your development?

Person 2: _____

Interviewer: I see, why is it important?

Person 2: _____

Interviewer: Thank you. And here we have another person. In your opinion, what is one *social* factor that helps in your development?

Person 3: _____

Interviewer: That's very interesting. Why do you think that is important?

Person 3: _____

(Continue alternating physical, emotional, mental, and social factors.)

Interviewer: Thank you very much ladies and gentlemen. That's all of our time for today. Do join us tomorrow for another exciting person-on-the-street interview. Take it away back at Station K.N.O.W.

Suggested Follow-Up:

1. What other factors are important that were not mentioned?
2. Which factors have contributed to your own growth and development?

Feelings About Growing

Concept:

Growing and developing follow a predictable sequence yet are unique for each individual.

General Behavioral Objective:

The student will be able to demonstrate an understanding of people growing and developing at different rates.

Domain: Affective   *Dimension:* Physical

Grade Level: Upper elementary

Specific Behavioral Objective:

In small groups, through role playing, the student will be able to share feelings about being "slower" or "faster" in developing.

Situation 1:

Tall girl being teased about her height.

Roles:

Tall Girl: You are taller than the other girls of your age. You feel that you are a "freak." You are very self-conscious and unhappy because you are tall.

Boy: You are only average in height. You wish you were as tall as _____, but you don't want anyone to know this. You enjoy teasing her about her height.

Girl: You are shorter than the other girls of your age. You wish you were as tall as _____ but don't want anyone to know this. You delight in teasing _____ about her height.

Situation 2:

Tall girl being teased about her height.

Roles:

Tall Girl: You are taller than the other girls of your age. Both of your parents are tall. You think it's great to be tall. Think of all the ways being tall is good, so that you can speak up when you are being teased. Tell the others that you are growing at your own rate just as they are.

Boy/Girl Roles: Same as Situation 1.

Situation 3:

Short boy being teased about his height.

Roles:

Short Boy: You are shorter than the other boys of your age. Your parents are both short. You wish that you would be tall but realize that you probably won't be. Tell the ones teasing you that: (1) you can't control your height any more than they can, (2) you are growing at the right rate for you, and (3) short people can be just as capable as tall people.

Boy: You are taller than the other boys your age. You feel awkward and uncomfortable being so tall. You enjoy teasing _____ because he's shorter.

Girl: You are taller than the other girls your age. You wish you were shorter. You enjoy teasing _____ because he's short.

Situation 4:

Short boy being teased about his height.

Roles:

Short Boy: You are shorter than the other boys your age. Your parents are tall and so are your older brothers and sisters. You are worried that you are going to be the "runt" of the family.

Boy: (Same as Situation 3)

Girl: You think it's very unfair for _____ to be teased about his height. You know that both of his parents and his older brothers and sisters are tall. Stick up for him. Use arguments like: What's so terrible about being short? With everyone in his family being tall, the chances are that he will be, too. Everyone grows at a different rate so his size is right for him.

Directions:

1. Other situations and roles can be written:
   a. overweight
   b. underweight
2. Role playing can be done in small groups or in class situation.

Suggested Follow-Up:

1. Discussion:
   a. How do you feel when you are teased about things you can't control?
   b. Why do we tease others?
2. Read roles of "teasers."
3. Write about personal feelings in being "faster" or "slower" in developing than friends are.
4. Read and discuss experiences without using names.

concept 3:

Protection and Promotion of Health Are Individual, Community, and International Responsibilities

Introduction to Concept — Lower Elementary Level

HAPPY'S DREAM

"Time for bed!" Happy's mother announced. "Here is a piece of cheese and a glass of juice. Eat them and then brush your teeth and crawl into bed."

The cheese was her very favorite kind and the juice washed down every tasty bite. Happy's head was already nodding. It had been a very busy day. As she crawled under the blankets she felt very good. She was still warm from her bath. Her tummy was full. She reached over and turned off the lamp. It wouldn't be long before she would be drifting into dreamland. "Today was fun," she thought to herself. "The teacher smiled and patted me on the head. It was fun playing

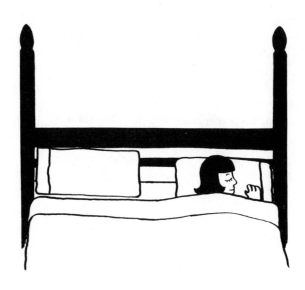

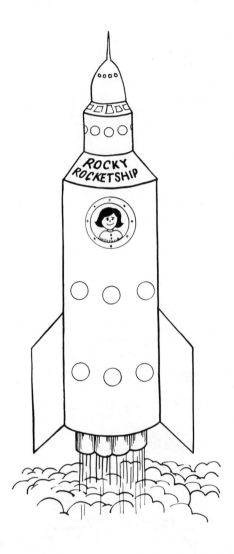

tag on the playground. I can run much faster than I used to . . . ."
ZZZZZZ. Happy was fast asleep.

It wasn't very long before she had the strange feeling that she was
flying through the air at a very high speed. She looked around and
saw that she was in a tiny room. When Happy looked out the window she saw nothing but the blue of the sky — and she felt frightened.
Then she heard a voice that sounded like it was coming from the
walls. "Don't be afraid," the voice said, "I am Rocky Rocketship
and I am taking you on a trip to far-off lands. Pretty soon you can

look into the "Super Seer" and see how some of the boys and girls in other places are living." Happy thought that would be lots of fun.

"Now!" said Rocky. Happy looked into the "Super Seer." She saw some things she did not expect to see. There were no boys and girls running and playing, going to school, sleeping in warm, clean, soft beds, or eating good food. Instead she saw that the families were huddled around a fire trying to keep warm. The children were crying

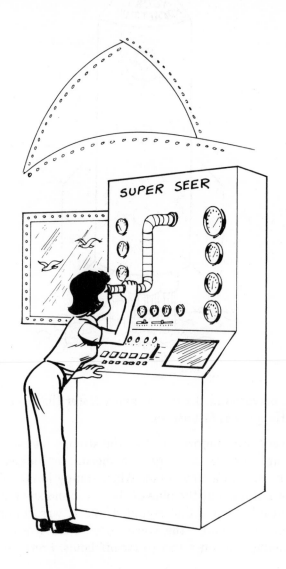

for food their parents could not give them — because there was none. Some of the people were sick and the others were trying to help them. It was a frightening sight to see and Happy felt badly. Rocky explained that there were millions of people just like that all over the world.

"I'm going to change course now and take you somewhere else," said Rocky. Soon Rocky told her to look into the "Super Seer" again. Happy saw a group of people living in a barren desert area. "They look like the American Indians," Happy said to Rocky. "They are," Rocky said, "but look a little closer." When she did, Happy noticed that they did not look like the pictures she had seen of the proud Indians. Again she noticed that they were very poor and their homes were not like hers. She also saw that there were many sick people among them. "Oh, the poor Indians," cried Happy, "and they live in *our* country!"

"We have one more place to go," announced Rocky, and away they flew in another direction. "Look now, Happy!" This time she saw some familiar places and she recognized that this was the town in which she lived. She was able to see down into a tiny home not too far from hers. The scene was almost the same as she had seen before — a family huddled around the fireplace with very little food to eat. The furniture was broken and the people's clothing was tattered and torn.

Happy started to cry. She had *never, ever* thought that there were people suffering right in her own town, her own country, and in other lands around the world. She had never really thought of anyone but herself and her own comfort.

"What can I do to help these people?" she asked Rocky.

"Why don't you ask your classmates when you go to school tomorrow?" he replied. "Maybe they can give you some suggestions."

Happy awakened suddenly and found that her pillow was wet. She really had been crying. Even though it was a dream, she knew that she would ask her classmates to help her discover ways she could help others to lead healthier, happier lives wherever they live.

If you were Happy's classmates, what might you tell her?

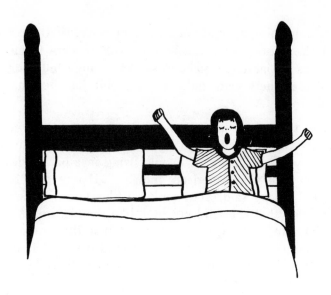

Helping-Hand Trip

Concept:

The protection and promotion of health are individual, community, and international responsibilities.

General Behavioral Objective:

The student will be able to identify ways to promote and protect the health of others.

Domain: Affective   *Dimension:* Physical, Social, Emotional

Grade Level: Lower elementary readers/nonreaders

Specific Behavioral Objective:

The student will be able to demonstrate values of caring for the needs of others by planning a "Helping Hand" trip.

Directions: (Teacher)

    1. Show pictures of people around the world.

      a. Use examples of people who have physical needs as well as people who are relatively well off.

2. Have each student make a pretend suitcase.
   a. Use one piece of manila construction paper folded in half and stapled on three sides.
   b. Attach handles to open side.
   c. Color as desired.
3. Provide magazines for nonreaders to cut up.

Directions: (Student)

1. Introduction:

   You all have marvelous imaginations! Today you are going to use yours to plan a pretend "Helping Hand" trip.

   You may choose to take this trip to another part of your own community (town, neighborhood), to another part of our country, or to another part of the world. You must plan what you are going to take on your trip. But there is one thing you must remember. *Everything you take on your trip in your suitcase must be helpful to the people you visit.*

   Think of ten things you would want to share with others where you are going. What you take may be both *things* (such as food or tools), and it may be *feelings* (such as love or honesty).

2. Nonreaders:

   a. You may use the magazines to cut out pictures of things you would like to share with others on your trip.
   b. If you cannot find something you want in the magazines, draw your own pictures on separate pieces of paper.
   c. Put each picture you find or draw into your suitcase. *Be sure you have no more than ten.*

3. Readers:

   a. Think of ten *things* or *feelings* you would like to share with others on your trip.
   b. Write each *thing* or *feeling* on separate pieces of paper and put them in your suitcase.

Suggested Follow-Up:

1. Have each pupil reveal and explain to the class:
   a. where he/she was going (community, other part of the country or world)

b. what is in his/her suitcase

c. how each item would be helpful to others

2. Play an elimination values-type game. One by one have student eliminate an item from his/her suitcase that he/she feels is of lesser value than those remaining. When they get down to one, have him/her reveal to the class that which they feel is most helpful to take and share with others.

Whose Responsibility Is It?

Concept:

The protection and promotion of health are individual, community, and international responsibilities.

General Behavioral Objective:

The student will be able to identify the responsibilities involved in the protection of health.

Domain: Cognitive   *Dimension:* All

Grade Level: Lower elementary

Specific Behavioral Objective:

Given a series of behaviors concerning the protection of health, the student will be able to identify who has the responsibility for each behavior by circling the correct word(s).

Directions: (Teacher)

1. Duplicate the "Whose Responsibility Is It?" worksheet (p. 85).

2. Read each statement or have the students complete the work on their own.

Directions: (Student)

1. Read each statement on your worksheet. If you think that what the statement says is your responsibility, circle the word "my." If you think it is a family responsibility, circle the word "family's." If you think it is the responsibility of the community in which you live, circle the word "community's." If you think that what the statement says is a responsibility of our country, circle the word "country's."

If you think that what is said is the responsibility of other nations of the world, circle the words "other countries'."

2. It is very important that you understand that *you may circle more than one answer after each statement.* Think! Whose responsibility is it?

Suggested Follow-Up:

1. Have students justify why they answer each statement as they did.
2. Have students draw a picture depicting:

  a. a way he/she can stay healthy.

  b. a way his/her family helps to keep him/her healthy.

  c. a way the community provides health protection.

  d. a way our country helps its citizens to be well.

  e. a way other countries can help those that have health problems.

WHOSE RESPONSIBILITY IS IT?

1. Throwing trash in the trash can.

   My   Family's   Community's   Country's   Other Countries'

2. Feeding starving people any place on earth.

   My   Family's   Community's   Country's   Other Countries'

3. Taking me to a doctor to get shots so I won't become sick.

   My   Family's   Community's   Country's   Other Countries'

4. Making laws to protect people's health.

   My   Family's   Community's   Country's   Other Countries'

5. Making sure I have pure water to drink.

   My   Family's   Community's   Country's   Other Countries'

6. Providing good schools for me.

   My   Family's   Community's   Country's   Other Countries'

7. Learning.

   My   Family's   Community's   Country's   Other Countries'

8. Having police and firefighters to protect me.

   My   Family's   Community's   Country's   Other Countries'

9. To see that I eat the right foods.

   My   Family's   Community's   Country's   Other Countries'

Health Helpers Puzzle/Report Card

Concept:

Protection and promotion of health are individual, community, and international responsibilities.

General Behavioral Objective:

The student will be able to identify the responsibilities involved in the protection of health.

Domain: Cognitive   *Dimension:* Physical

Grade Level: Lower elementary

Specific Behavioral Objective:

By solving the "Health Helpers" puzzle, the student will be able to identify people in the community who help to protect one's own physical health.

Directions: (Teacher)

    1. Duplicate the "Health Helpers" puzzle (p. 86–87).
    2. Duplicate the "Health Helper Report Card" (p. 88).

Directions: (Student)

On worksheet.

Suggested Follow-Up:

    1. Have students evaluate their own health behaviors on the Health Helper Report Card.
    2. Make a class collage-type bulletin board of pictures of health helpers in the community. Students can cut out pictures from magazines and paste them on construction paper. Then all individual projects can be grouped together on the bulletin board.

HEALTH HELPERS PUZZLE

Directions:

From this list of health helpers, choose the correct word or words to fill in the blanks in each sentence.

trash collector	fireman
doctor	policeman
school nurse	custodian
dentist	teacher

1. The _ _ _ _ _ _ helps keep my teeth healthy.

2. The _ _ _ _ _ _ helps me to keep from being sick and helps me to get well when I am sick.

3. The _ _ _ _ _ _ _ _ _ _ _ _ _ helps to keep my neighborhood clean.

4. My _ _ _ _ _ _ _ helps me to learn how to stay healthy.

5. The _ _ _ _ _ _ _ _ _ is a friend who helps protect me from harm.

6. Our _ _ _ _ _ _ _ _ _ _ helps keep our school clean and safe.

7. A _ _ _ _ _ _ _ helps to prevent and put out fires.

8. The _ _ _ _ _ _ _ _ _ _ _ helps me when I become sick or hurt at school.

Litterbugs

Concept:

Protection and promotion of health are individual, community, and international responsibilities.

General Behavioral Objective:

The student will be able to describe the effects of littering on the health of the community.

Domain: Cognitive   *Dimension:* Physical

Grade Level: Lower elementary-readers/nonreaders

Specific Behavioral Objectives:

Nonreaders: After drawing a picture of an imaginary litterbug, the student will be able to describe verbally how litterbugs hurt a community.

Readers: Given verbs beginning with the letters in the word LITTERBUG, the student will be able to describe in writing some of the behaviors of a litterbug that hurt a community.

MY HEALTH HELPER REPORT CARD

My name is _____

(Circle the correct answer)

I have had my teeth checked in the past year.

Yes No

I have had a vaccination for measles.

Yes No

I help keep my yard clean.

Yes No Sometimes

I try to practice good health habits.

Yes No Sometimes

I never talk to strangers on the street.

Yes No Sometimes

I am careful when using fire in any way.

Yes No Sometimes

I stay home from school when I am sick.

Yes No Sometimes

I pick up trash in the school and on the playground.

Yes No Sometimes

I am a HEALTH HELPER.

Yes No Sometimes

Directions: (Teacher)

Nonreaders:

1. Students draw a picture of what they think a litterbug looks like.
2. Each student shows picture to the class and describes one thing a litterbug does to hurt a community.

Directions: (Teacher)

Readers:

1. Duplicate the "Litterbugs" worksheet (p. 89).
2. Students write a description of one behavior of a litterbug for each verb.

LITTERBUGS

L EAVE

I GNORE

T HROW

T AKE

E MPTY

R IP

B REAK

U SE

G IVE

Suggested Follow-Up:

Nonreaders:

1. Role play the events in the one-day life of one of the following agents of littering:

a. I am a package of gum.

b. I am a can of pop.

c. I am a candy bar.

d. I am a lunch bag.

In the role play describe what they look like, how they feel, what they do, and how they got to be called "litter."

2. Plan and act out a skit called "The Day the Litterbug Came to Town."

Readers:

1. In small groups, write and act out a skit entitled "I Love Litterbugs." They could use characters of their choice or one of these suggested:

ROTTEN RAT

DIZZY DISEASE

ANGIE ACCIDENT

WACKY RACOON

FILTHY FLY

ACTIVE ANT

"We Care!"

Concept:

Protection and promotion of health are individual, community, and international responsibilities.

General Behavioral Objective:

The student will be able to identify ways to promote and protect others in the community.

Domain: Affective   *Dimension:* Physical

Grade Level: Lower elementary

Specific Behavioral Objective:

The student will be able to demonstrate the concern for the health and welfare of others in the community by providing a food and clothing "We Care!" package for a needy family.

Directions: (Teacher)

1. With help from a local church or other community organization get a list of food and clothing needs for a local family, or

2. Respond to a newspaper request for aid to a needy family.

3. Collect, box, and transport the "We Care!" package to the organization or the family, as appropriate.

Directions: (Students)

1. Introduction:

   All of us need things from time to time. Sometimes our needs are great. Sometimes they are small. Usually when we *really* need something we are able to get it. For example, when you need a new pair of shoes, someone will usually buy them for you. Or if your family needs more milk, someone will go to the store and get it.

   Did you ever stop to think that there are some families in our own community who, because of illness, fire, tornado, or other reasons, do not have enough money to buy food and clothing? I know of one such family that needs help. Can any of you suggest what we can do, as a class, to help? Who can tell me what the word "care" means? How about the word "package?" What do you think a "care package" is? Do you suppose that our class can organize a "We Care!" package for the needy family?

2. Procedure:

   a. You will each be a member of one of these committees for our project:
      1. Canned food committee
      2. Nearly-new clothing committee
      3. Money-collecting committee
      4. Packing committee

   b. The duties of each committee are as follows:
      1. Canned food committee—Try to encourage classmates to bring in a variety of canned food. Make sure there are foods from all four food groups (review).
      2. Nearly-new clothing committee—Encourage classmates to donate clothing that is outgrown but not worn-out. Announce the sizes needed to the class.
      3. Money-collecting committee—Ask classmates to donate money so that fresh food can be purchased just before the "care package" is delivered.
      4. Packing committee—Bring in strong boxes and pack them with the food and clothing.

3. Even though each of you is only on one committee, you may help the other committees by your donations.

4. See if we can fill at least one "We Care!" package in three days.

Suggested Follow-Up:

1. Explain the feelings they have from having people less fortunate than they.
2. Explain how they would feel if something happened to their family that stopped all money from coming in.

---

concept 3:

Protection and Promotion of Health Are Individual, Community, and International Responsibilities.

Introduction to Concept — Upper Elementary Level

HARRY HOTSHOT

Harry Hotshot is a young man just about your age. He fancied himself as being a great athlete, and indeed he was quite skilled in almost all kinds of sports. His great love was basketball. Since he was quite tall for his age, he played the center position on his Saturday morning recreational team, the Tigers. Harry should have been the real leader of the team, but because he was always boasting about how good he was, his teammates turned him off.

The Tigers were tied for first place with the Bearcats. The championship game was scheduled to be played the next Saturday. Harry told everyone that the Tigers would beat the Bearcats and that he would be the high scorer in the game.

When Saturday came, the school gym was crowded with parents and fans from all over town. They were all filled with excitement.

Much to Harry's surprise the Bearcats got the tip-off, even though he was taller than the opposing center. From that moment on, it was all downhill for the Tigers. Harry "hogged" the ball — he just wouldn't pass it off to his teammates, even though they were sometimes in better position to shoot the ball then he was. He dribbled the ball all by himself only to have one of the Bearcats steal it away or block his shot. The Bearcats didn't seem to have a big star. Everyone seemed to be scoring an almost equal number of points.

When the final buzzer sounded ending the game, the Bearcats had won. Harry had the most points in the game, but his team had lost.

Why do you think the Bearcats beat the Tigers?

Have you ever thought seriously about the word "teamwork?" Who can tell us what it means?

Teamwork is when a group of people puts aside its own selfish interests and works together to reach a goal that is important to all members of the group.

Why would Harry have been a more valuable member of his team if he had practiced teamwork?

We are all members of different kinds of teams all our lives. The success of those teams depends upon how well the members work together. Let's see if you can recognize some kinds of teamwork that help contribute to the health and well-being of people.

I will read a series of statements. If you think that the statement describes real teamwork that helps people, make a fist with your thumb pointing up. If you think the statement describes selfishness that does not help people, make a fist and point your thumb down.

Note to teacher: You may wish to discuss each statement after the vote.

1. Your family and you work together to protect the health of each member.
2. When you are sick, you stay home from school.
3. You throw trash on the ground wherever you happen to be.
4. The doctors, nurses, and other people in the hospital work to make people well.
5. The police and firemen protect the citizens from harm.
6. A large factory dumps its wastes into a nearby stream from which a town down the river gets its water supply.
7. You leave lights and electrical appliances on when they are not necessary.
8. Your family contributes money to the many health agencies that help others (American Cancer Society, Heart Association, United Funds, UNICEF, Red Cross, Lung Association, Muscular Dystrophy, March of Dimes, etc.).

9. You decide to smoke because your best friend does.
10. The United States government spends money for health research.
11. The United States contributes to the World Health Organization.
12. You are/aren't concerned when others in your community do not have enough to eat.
13. You would rather play pranks on people on Halloween than collect money for UNICEF.
14. One country overfishes areas of the ocean.
15. When disaster strikes an area of the world, other countries send help.

I have a riddle for you to solve. It concerns the subject we have been discussing. If you know the answer after I read it, point your thumb up but do not tell anyone.

THE RIDDLE

I'm thinking of a word that is short and sweet
That without many people, it would not be complete
It starts with a "T" and ends with a "K"
It's important to health, in every way.

If your thumb is up, call out your answer together. If you said "teamwork," you were right!

It All Depends on Me

Concept:

Protection and promotion of health are individual, community, and international responsibilities.

General Behavioral Objective:

The student will be able to explain ways that the health of others is dependent upon his/her own well-being.

Domain: Affective   *Dimension:* Mental

Grade Level: Upper elementary

Specific Behavioral Objective:

After completing the last lines in the stanzas of a poem, the student will be able to explain verbally ways to personally contribute to the health and welfare of others.

Directions: (Teacher)

1. Students work individually or in dyads.
2. Put each stanza on a clear acetate, or
3. Read each stanza of "It All Depends on Me" (pp. 95-96).
4. Set a time limit for completing the last line.
5. Discuss questions posed after each stanza.

Directions: (Students)

1. On each transparency is a stanza from the poem, "It All Depends on Me."
2. Part of the last line of each stanza is missing.
3. You will have _____ minutes to complete the line. Make the last word of your line rhyme with the last word of the previous line. Write your last line on a piece of paper.
4. Read the stanza with your last line.
5. Verbally answer the questions at the end of each stanza.

Suggested Follow-Up:

1. Complete the stem sentence:
   I am an important person to everyone in the world because . . .

IT ALL DEPENDS ON ME

Stanza 1:

> Health is important to everyone
> Wherever they live under the sun.
> In all nations, large or small,
> To live well is . . .

(Suggestion to teacher: ". . . the goal of all")

Discussion: "How can I help — what can I do to help people in other countries to improve their health?"

Stanza 2:

> Here in our country proud and strong,
> It seems that health problems don't belong.

Yet look about you and you'll agree,
That everyone is not . . .

(Suggestion to teacher: ". . . healthy as can be" or
". . . entirely free")

Discussion: "How can I help — what can I do to help solve some of the health problems in our country?"

Stanza 3:

Living conditions may not be all that good,
Here in my town or my neighborhood.
Hunger, stress, disease, crime, even pollution
Demand that I help . . .

(Suggestion to teacher: ". . . to find a solution")

Discussion: "How can I help — what can I do to help improve the health of my community?"

Stanza 4:

I will work very hard to take care of me
Physically, mentally, and socially,
So my town, my country, and my world will be
Better places for all . . .

(Suggestion to teacher: ". . . to live healthily")

Discussion: "How can I help — what can I do to improve my own health?"

Community Helper Word Search

Concept:

Protection and promotion of health are individual, community, and international responsibilities.

General Behavioral Objective:

The student will be able to identify people in the community who work to protect and promote good health.

Domain: Cognitive   *Dimension:* Mental

Grade Level: Upper elementary

Specific Behavioral Objective:

The student will be able to identify in writing some people in the community who contribute to the protection and promotion of his/her health by solving a word search.

Directions: (Teacher)

1. Duplicate the Word Search Puzzle (p. 98).
2. Students work individually to discover some people or groups of people in the community that help to protect and promote his/her health.
3. Key: police, firemen, doctor, nurse, dentist, farmer, food inspector, sanitary engineer, teacher, lifeguard, safety patrol, health department, lawmakers, trash collector, and custodian.

Suggested Follow-Up:

1. Write a brief description of how each of the people or group of people discovered in the puzzle contributes to his/her own health.
2. Pantomine one of the jobs listed and have class guess which one it is.
3. Write and act out a skit portraying what life in the community would be like if one of those people or groups of people did not exist.

WORD SEARCH PUZZLE

People In Our Community Who Help Protect My Health

Directions: There are many people and groups of people right here in our community that help you to stay healthy. Follow the directions carefully and see how many you can discover.

1. This is a word search puzzle. As you find the people or group of people that help you, circle it and write it down in the space provided on page 2 of the worksheet. There are 15 possible answers.
2. You may find the words across, backward, up, down, or diagonally. Good luck!

B	E	R	O	T	C	E	P	S	N	I	D	C	O	F	T
D	S	L	A	W	M	A	K	E	R	S	D	E	O	A	R
C	R	P	L	A	S	S	F	M	D	T	E	N	E	R	A
G	U	T	F	V	F	I	M	D	Z	O	N	Y	D	M	S
T	N	E	M	T	R	A	P	E	D	H	T	L	A	E	H
E	H	J	Q	E	N	K	O	E	F	R	I	I	X	R	C
A	N	I	M	U	C	Q	L	Y	N	W	S	F	U	R	O
C	C	E	Z	U	P	H	I	R	G	K	T	E	L	C	L
H	N	O	V	R	O	T	C	O	D	D	P	G	L	W	L
E	J	I	I	J	G	K	E	J	L	X	T	U	B	S	E
R	O	L	O	R	T	A	P	Y	T	E	F	A	S	B	C
H	G	B	N	A	I	D	O	T	S	U	C	R	M	Y	T
Q	V	A	K	I	Z	A	W	M	H	A	E	D	X	F	O
S	A	N	I	T	A	R	Y	E	N	G	I	N	E	E	R

PEOPLE IN OUR COMMUNITY WHO HELP
PROTECT MY HEALTH

List here those people or groups that you have discovered in the
Word Search Puzzle.

1. _____   9. _____

2. _____   10. _____

3. _____   11. _____

4. _____   12. _____

5. _____   13. _____

6. _____   14. _____

7. _____   15. _____

8. _____

Partner Interview

Concept:

Protection and promotion of health are individual, community, and international responsibilities.

General Behavioral Objective:

The student will be able to cite ways to protect emotional health.

Domain: Cognitive   *Dimension:* Emotional

Grade Level: Upper elementary

Specific Behavioral Objective:

Working in dyads, the student will be able to discover the ways other people relieve tensions by interviewing the partner.

Directions: (Teacher)

1. Introduce by explaining that everyone gets upset by events that happen to them from time to time. In order to keep emotionally and mentally healthy, we need to deal with the problems through actions. Different people do different things to relieve their tensions.
2. Divide class into dyads.
3. Conduct interviews.
4. Make a report of findings.
5. List events and actions on the chalkboard.

Directions: (Student)

1. Make two columns on a sheet of paper. Head one: Events, head the other: Actions.
2. Meet with partner.
3. Interview partner:
   a. What has happened that upsets you?
   b. What do you do when this happens?
4. Record answers.

Suggested Follow-Up:

1. Using the master list generated by the class, students determine if each is a physical, mental, or social means of relieving tensions.
2. Using the master list, students indicate why they think each means of relieving tensions is effective or ineffective.

3. Draw two cartoons, one depicting their opinion of an effective way to deal with a specific tension-provoking problem, and the other showing an ineffective way to deal with the problem. Title the cartoons with a statement of the problem (example: name-calling).
4. Complete the following stem-sentences:
   a. My family helps me to protect my emotional health by . . .
   b. My community helps me to protect my emotional health by providing . . .

The Good Guys/The Bad Guys Skit

Concept:

Promotion and protection of health are individual, community, and international responsibilities.

General Behavioral Objective:

The pupil will be able to demonstrate ways to promote social health.

Domain: Affective   *Dimension:* Social

Grade Level: Upper elementary

Specific Behavioral Objective:

After selecting a situation describing a specific behavior, the students, in groups of four, will be able to demonstrate ways of promoting and hurting social relationships by developing a skit.

Directions: (Teacher)

1. Prepare a box with a slit in the lid large enough for a child's hand to reach in.
2. Label the box "THE GOOD GUYS/THE BAD GUYS."
3. On 3 × 5 cards describe a variety of social behaviors. Put the cards in the box. Suggested behaviors:
   a. teasing someone who makes a mistake
   b. laughing when someone gets hurt
   c. ignoring a new student in the room
   d. ganging up on a person who is different than you
   e. taking something that doesn't belong to you
   f. fighting with your brother or sister
   g. blaming someone for something you did

h. cheating when playing a game

i . lying to your parents

4. Duplicate directions for each group.

5. Organize students into groups of four.

Directions: (Students)

1. How you get along with other people is called your SOCIAL RELATIONSHIPS. Much of your happiness in life depends upon these relationships with other people.

   There are many ways you can help to improve or hurt others' feelings about you. At the same time there are many ways you can help or hurt the way you feel about yourself or the way others feel about themselves.

   Today we are going to play a game called "The Good Guys/ The Bad Guys."

2. One member of your group will come to the Good Guys/ Bad Guys box and take one card from it. Go back to your group without telling other groups what is on your card.

3. Quietly read the situation to your group members.

4. Two of your group members will be "Bad Guys" and the other two will be "Good Guys."

5. Your job is to make up a skit about the situation. The "Bad Guys" will show how they would act in that situation, and the "Good Guys" will show how they would act.

Suggested Follow-Up:

1. Assign the observing groups to determine:

   a. what the behavior was

   b. who the "Good Guys" and who the "Bad Guys" were

2. After each group has performed, each small group makes up a new situation and writes it on a piece of paper. Repeat the skits using one chosen from the class-derived situations.

Earthquake!

Concept:

Protection and promotion of health are individual, community, and international responsibilities.

General Behavioral Objective:

The student will be able to demonstrate an understanding of the mutual responsibility among nations for the health and welfare of others.

Domain: Affective   *Dimension:* Physical

Grade Level: Upper elementary

Specific Behavioral Objective:

In small groups, the students, representing a variety of countries, will be able to describe in writing the kind of physical aid that could be provided in the event of an earthquake in a make-believe country.

Directions: (Teacher)

Note: This lesson may be planned as a correlated learning experience with geography and/or social studies.

1. Organize students into groups of no more than four.
2. Make up a name for a make-believe country such as Terranonfirma, San Miguel, or Terrabella.
3. Place the names of several real countries from a variety of geographical locations in a box.
4. Each group draws the name of a country from the box.

Introduction:

An important newsflash has just been made on television and radio! The tiny country of San Miguel has suffered a terrible earthquake. The first reports from a pilot in a helicopter say that much of this beautiful Central American country has been destroyed. Thousands of people have been hurt and hundreds are thought to be dead. Homes and buildings in the villages and cities have been wrecked and lines of communication have been broken off.

You have been called to this meeting as representatives of your country to forget your own differences and plan how you are going to help the people of San Miguel.

Directions: (Students)

1. Your small group represents the country whose name you drew from the box.
2. Your job is to come up with a list of things and people from your country that you can send to help the people of San Miguel.

3. In order to do the job, you will have to use the resource materials in the room to better understand what products and natural resources are available in your country and what skills your people have that could be helpful.
4. Three people in your group will be the chief researchers and one person will be both a researcher and a report writer.
5. Do a good job because the lives of many people are in your hands. Good luck!

Suggested Follow-Up:

1. Have students read the group report to the class. Have them justify how each of the products or people they are sending to San Miguel will be helpful.
2. As a conclusion, have each student complete this stem sentence:
   I believe that the big idea from this learning has been that . . .

---

concept 4:

The Potential for Hazards and Accidents Exists, Whatever the Environment

---

Introduction to Concept — Lower Elementary Level

ANGIE ACCIDENT

To the teacher:

Before introducing the concept, make a hand puppet of the character "Angie Accident" (p. 104).

Introduction:

"Hi there! I'm Angie Accident! Do you know what my last name means? Do you know that I cause more boys and girls your age to be hurt and to die than anything else? Have I been a part of your life this week? How about in this past year? Is there any way you could have prevented me from happening? How?

I don't just *happen.* I am *caused* by something *you* or *someone else does or does not do.* Think about when I was in your life last. Was I caused by something you or someone else *did* or something you or someone else *did not do* that could have prevented me from happening?

Since I am caused by people and no person is always perfectly in control of his thinking, his feelings, and what he is doing, I will always be in your life and everyone else's.

What you need to do is to cut down on the number of times I appear in your life — especially the number of times I cause you to be badly hurt."

Angie Accident would like to teach you to recognize the different ways that she can hurt or kill you and the people around you. Also, Angie wants you to know what you can do to keep her out of your life most of the time. She will examine the feelings you have before and after she enters your life. Angie has many activities planned to remind you and your friends to "think safety" all of the time.

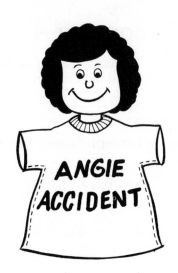

Angie's Safety Rules

Concept:

The potential for hazards and accidents exists, whatever the environment.

General Behavioral Objective:

The student will be able to describe ways to promote safety awareness in self and in others.

Domain: Cognitive/Psychomotor   *Dimension:* Physical

Grade Level: Lower elementary

Specific Behavioral Objective:

1. The students, in total class discussion, will be able to suggest a series of safety rules, each one beginning with the letters in Angie Accident.

Directions: (Student)

1. Think of some safety rules that will keep you from getting hurt or even from getting killed. Make your safety rule begin with one of the letters in Angie Accident's name. Here is an example of one rule:

Always look both ways before you cross the street.

N . . .

G . . .

I . . .

E . . .

A . . .

C . . .

C . . .

I . . .

D . . .

E . . .

N . . .

T . . .

Suggested Follow-Up:

1. Choose one of the rules that you would like to show in a picture you will draw and color.
2. Take one piece of manila paper from the table, and
3. Color the picture. Make it look as neat and colorful as you can.

4. Print the safety rule on your picture.

5. When you are finished, hang your picture on the ANGIE ACCIDENT bulletin board.

Helpful Fires, Harmful Fires

Concept:

The potential for hazards and accidents exists, whatever the environment.

General Behavioral Objective:

The student will be able to discuss ways fire can be both helpful and harmful.

Domain: Cognitive   *Dimension:* Social

Grade Level: Lower elementary

Specific Behavioral Objectives:

1. Through class discussion, the student will be able to generate a list of ways fire is (a) helping the family at home, (b) helping students at school.

2. Through class discussion, the student will be able to identify ways that fire could be harmful at home and at school.

Directions: (Teacher)

1. Prepare tagboard strips with magnetic tape on back. Preprint eight strips: HELPS, FIRE HELPS, HOME, SCHOOL, HARMS, FIRE HARMS, HOME, SCHOOL.

2. Use "helps" and "harms" for learning the meaning of the terms. Verbally give examples of people or things that help or harm. Have students point to or say the term that applies.

3. Place the other tagboard headings on the chalkboard. As the helps and harms are generated, they can be listed under the proper heading. If class aides are available, additional labels can be printed and placed on chalkboard.

	Fire Helps			*Fire Harms*	
Home		*School*	*Home*		*School*

I'm A Fire

Concept:

The potential for hazards and accidents exists, whatever the environment.

General Behavioral Objective:

The student will be able to demonstrate ways that fire can be both helpful and harmful.

Domain: Psychomotor   *Dimension:* Social

Grade Level: Lower elementary

Specific Behavioral Objective:

Individually, the student will be able to role play "I am a harmful fire" or "I am a helpful fire" in either a school or home environment.

Directions: (Teacher)

1. Use the lists generated by the class in "Helpful Fires, Harmful Fires."
2. Pass out a label to a student. If a nonreader, whisper what help or harm is to be role played.

Directions: (Student)

1. Use sounds and motions to show the kind of fire you are.
2. Other students can ask questions which can be answered by "yes" or "no."
3. The student who guesses correctly takes your place.

Suggested Follow-Up:

1. Alternative activity using hand or stick puppets.
   a. Two students: a questioner and a "fire."
   b. Dialogue:
      1) "What kind of fire are you?"
      2) "I'm a helpful fire."
      3) "Are you at home or at school?"
      4) "I'm used in both places."
      5) "What are you used for?"
      6) "I'm used to make meals."
      7) "You're a gas stove."

Walking to Safety

Concept:

The potential for hazards and accidents exists, whatever the environment.

General Behavioral Objective:

The student will be able to demonstrate ways to escape the effects of fire.

Domain: Psychomotor   *Dimension:* Physical

Grade Level: Lower elementary

Specific Behavioral Objective:

After tracing the fire drill routes established in the school, the student is able to demonstrate the ability to evacuate the school building safely from each location in the school where she/he might be.

Directions: (Teacher)

1. Discuss the importance to everyone's physical safety of knowing what to do in case of fire and then being able to do it properly.
2. Have entire class walk through the fire drill procedure and routes from the:
   a. classroom
   b. cafeteria
   c. auditorium
   d. library
   e. gymnasium
   f. girls' and boys' lavatories

Suggested Follow-Up:

1. Repeat activity for a tornado alert.

I Can Help Prevent Fire Accidents

Concept:

The potential for hazards and accidents exists, whatever the environment.

General Behavioral Objective:

The student will be able to explain how people can prevent fires from happening.

Domain: Cognitive   *Dimension:* Physical

Grade Level: Lower elementary

Specific Behavioral Objective:

On the worksheet provided, the pupil will be able to distinguish between good rules and bad rules for fire accident prevention by responding to the situations.

Directions: (Teacher)

1. Duplicate the "I Can Help Prevent Fire Accidents" worksheet (p. 110).
2. For primary pupils, read each statement.
3. Students circle the correct answer.

Suggested Follow-Up:

1. Repeat rules; students give reasons for their answers.
2. Students suggest other rules that would help to prevent fire accidents.

I CAN HELP PREVENT FIRE ACCIDENTS WORKSHEET

Directions:

Here is a list of rules.

If it is a good rule and will help prevent fire accidents, circle Yes, Yes!

If it is not a good rule and might help to cause a fire accident, circle No, No!

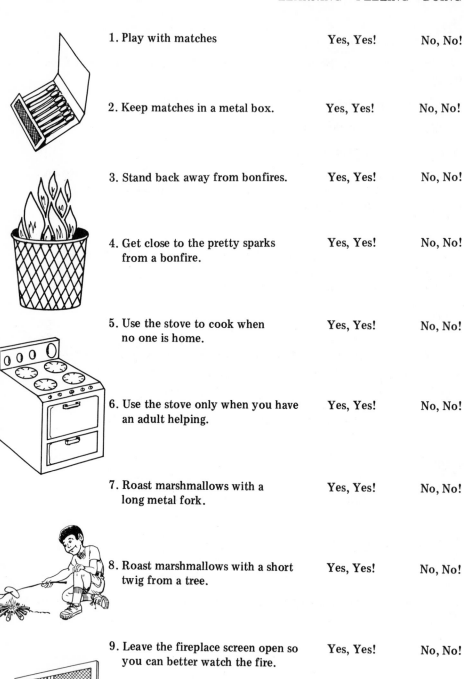

1. Play with matches   Yes, Yes!   No, No!

2. Keep matches in a metal box.   Yes, Yes!   No, No!

3. Stand back away from bonfires.   Yes, Yes!   No, No!

4. Get close to the pretty sparks   Yes, Yes!   No, No!
   from a bonfire.

5. Use the stove to cook when   Yes, Yes!   No, No!
   no one is home.

6. Use the stove only when you have   Yes, Yes!   No, No!
   an adult helping.

7. Roast marshmallows with a   Yes, Yes!   No, No!
   long metal fork.

8. Roast marshmallows with a short   Yes, Yes!   No, No!
   twig from a tree.

9. Leave the fireplace screen open so   Yes, Yes!   No, No!
   you can better watch the fire.

10. Make sure the fireplace screen is   Yes, Yes!   No, No!
    closed when there is a fire.

Station Learning

To the teacher:

One method that is particularly effective for students of all ages is Station Learning. This can be done in any subject area to accomplish a variety of related objectives in any given concept. When utilizing this method, the teacher truly serves as a facilitator as students are actively involved in their learning.

To carry out Station Learning efficiently, a great deal of thoughtful preparation must be done. The teacher must preplan:

1. the concept to be utilized,
2. the general area of the concept to be emphasized based upon student needs (general behavioral objectives),
3. the meaningful specific behaviors desired to accomplish the general behavioral objectives,
4. how to physically set up the learning stations in the room,
5. how to organize students so that each will be able to visit every station, and
6. the provision of all learning materials and resources needed by the students.

Any concept in health education lends itself beautifully to this type of learning. One thing that must be remembered, however, is that station learning is not just "fun and games." Even though some of the objectives may be reached through "games," ALL LEARNING MUST BE PURPOSEFUL.

As far as the physical set-up in the room for learning stations is concerned, the teacher alone must decide what is best, based upon what is available. Desks may be grouped together or tables with chairs may be used to make up a station. It is suggested that the various stations be scattered about the room to minimize the noise interference. Each station should be identified by a number or another meaningful symbol so that students will know where to move to next.

The students will visit the various learning stations in groups, although the learning to be accomplished at each station can be either a group or an individual endeavor. The group numbers ought not to exceed four or five. Consequently, the number of learning stations needed will be determined by the number of students in the class. The teacher must judge how many stations are to be visited in any given period of time and what, if any, the time limitation will be for each. (It must be remembered that more time will be needed for some students and less for others, so each must be accommodated.) It is further suggested that the teacher have a desk or table set up somewhere in the midst of the stations so that he/she is available for both facilitation and evaluation of the learning activities.

Supplies and resource materials must be made available to students either at each learning station or in a general area of the room. The learning experiences themselves, however, should be provided at the various stations with written directions, so that the students can readily read, understand, and perform the required behavior.

In this concept, at the lower elementary level, the preceding sample lessons are designed for regular classroom implementation. The ones which follow are designed for Station Learning. In both cases, the learning focuses on fire safety. It is hoped that these examples will help trigger your thoughts as to how you can design Station Learning experiences in other general areas of safety education, for any other concept of health education or for all other subject matter areas.

STATION #1: THE "?"

Concept:

The potential for hazards and accidents exists, whatever the environment.

General Behavioral Objective:

The student will be able to demonstrate an understanding of what to do in case of fire.

Domain: Cognitive   *Dimension:* Physical

Grade Level: Lower elementary

Specific Behavioral Objective:

After completing and identifying a dot-to-dot picture of a fireman, the student will be able to explain what to do in case of fire by completing a stem sentence.

Directions: (Teacher)

    1. Duplicate copies of The "?" Worksheet (p. 113).
    2. Prepare one copy of Directions for Station #1. Dry mount copy on a manila file folder.

Directions for Station #1:

    1. Take a copy of The "?" Worksheet.

    2. Draw a straight line from one number to the next until you have completed the picture. You now have a picture of a person who helps us when we need him.

3. Answer Questions 2 and 3 on the worksheet.

4. Color the picture.

5. Put your name on the worksheet and give it to your teacher.

6. You are now ready to go to Station #2.

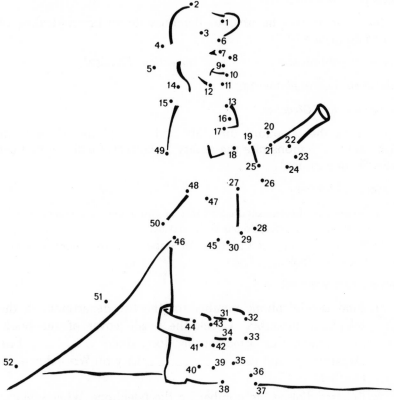

2. Circle the right answer.

   This friendly helper is a:

   Policeman   Fireman   Nurse   Garbageman

3. Give as many answers as you can to this sentence:

   If my house was on fire, I would . . . .

   a. _____

   b. _____

   c. _____

   d. _____

STATION #2: I WANT TO REPORT A FIRE

Concept:

The potential for hazards and accidents exists, whatever the environment.

General Behavioral Objective:

The student will be able to demonstrate an understanding of what to do in case of fire.

Domain: Psychomotor   *Dimension:* Physical

Grade Level: Lower elementary

Specific Behavioral Objective:

By using the telephone directory and a telephone, the student will be able to demonstrate the ability to correctly dial the number of the fire department.

Directions: (Teacher)

1. Secure two disconnected telephones or two extension telephones and a local phone directory to put at the station.
2. Prepare one copy of Directions for Station #2. Dry mount copy on a manila file folder.

Directions for Station #2.

1. Find the telephone number for the fire department in the telephone directory. Check the inside cover of the book; look under Fire Emergencies; look under _____ Fire Department, and under _____, City of. Write down the number.
2. Practice dialing the number on the telephone. When you can do it without looking at the written number, have the teacher check you out.
3. With a partner, practice reporting a fire.

   a. Your neighbor's house is on fire.

   b. A car is on fire in front of your house.
4. As the person playing the fire department, ask these questions:

   a. What is the address where the fire is?

   b. What is burning?

   c. Is it inside or outside?

   d. What kind of fire is it?

e. What is your name?

f. What is your telephone number?

5. You are now ready to go to Station #3.

STATION #3: DRAW THE WORD

Concept:

The potential for hazards and accidents exists, whatever the environment.

General Behavioral Objective:

The student will be able to demonstrate an understanding of the vocabulary related to fire safety.

Domain: Cognitive   *Dimension:* Mental

Grade Level: Lower elementary

Specific Behavioral Objective:

The student will be able to demonstrate an understanding of fire safety vocabulary by drawing pictures of specific words.

Directions: (Teacher)

1. Reproduce copies of "Draw the Word" Worksheet (p. 116).
2. Prepare one copy of Directions for Station #3. Dry mount copy on a manila file folder.

Directions: (Student)

1. Take one copy of "Draw the Word" Worksheet.

2. Complete the Worksheet.

3. Put the finished Worksheet in the "Done" box at your station.

4. You are now ready to go to Station #4.

STATION #4: FIRE SAFETY CROSSWORD PUZZLE

Concept:

The potential for hazards and accidents exists, whatever the environment.

General Behavioral Objective:

The student will be able to demonstrate an understanding of the vocabulary related to fire safety.

Draw The Word Worksheet

Directions:

Here are some words we use often when we speak about fires. Some of these are two words, others are one word with two syllables. After seeing the example given in number 1, see if you can draw pictures of the other words.

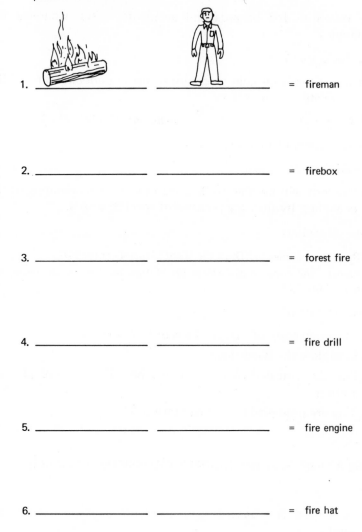

1. _____ _____ = fireman

2. _____ _____ = firebox

3. _____ _____ = forest fire

4. _____ _____ = fire drill

5. _____ _____ = fire engine

6. _____ _____ = fire hat

Domain: Cognitive   *Dimension:* Mental

Grade Level: Lower elementary

Specific Behavioral Objective:

The student will be able to demonstrate an understanding of fire safety vocabulary by completing a crossword puzzle.

Directions: (Teacher)

    1. Reproduce copies of the Fire Safety Crossword Puzzle (p. 118).

    2. Key for Puzzle:

ACROSS	*DOWN*
3. Firemen	1. Burn
5. Flame	2. Fireplace
7. Smoke	4. Matches
8. Fires	6. Accident
10. Fire drills	9. Alarm

    3. Prepare a copy of Directions for Station #4. Dry mount copy on a manila file folder.

Directions for Station #4:

1. Take one copy of the Fire Safety Crossword Puzzle.

2. Work alone or with a partner.

3. When you finish, take it to the teacher for it to be checked.

4. If all words are correct, you are now ready to move to Station #5.

Name _____

FIRE SAFETY CROSSWORD PUZZLE

Directions:

Read the clues given below the puzzle. The number of blocks will tell you how many letters are in the word. All of the words are about fire and fire safety.

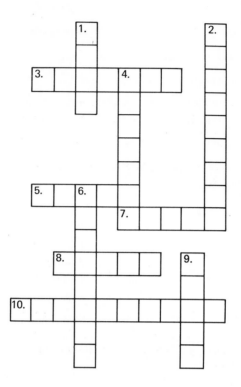

ACROSS

3. These people come when we report a fire.

5. What a fire has which is RED HOT!

7. This will pour out of a burning house.

8. At times these hurt and at times they help.

10. We have these at school so we will know what to do in case of fire.

DOWN

1. Fire will do this to your hand if you touch it.

2. The screen should always be closed if you have a fire in this place.

4. The objects that can cause fires if children play with them.

6. What we call it when a fire starts and we don't know what caused it.

9. If there is a fire at school, someone will pull the handle on this.

STATION #5: FLAME GAME[5]

Concept:

The potential for hazards and accidents exists, whatever the environment.

General Behavioral Objective:

The student will be able to explain fire safety rules.

Domain: Cognitive   *Dimension:* Mental

Grade Level: Lower elementary

Specific Behavioral Objective:

The student will be able to explain a variety of fire safety rules by playing the Flame card game.

Directions: (Teacher)

1. Prepare Flame Game Cards and Direction Sheet (pp. 120–121).
    a. Use heavy tagboard.
    b. Make 4 cards of each of the 12 pictures and 1 Flame card — 49 cards in the game.
    c. Color the pictures. Print the safety rules.
    d. Laminate the cards and the Direction Sheet with mylar film or clear contact paper.
2. Put a supply of blank cards at the station.
3. Prepare a copy of Directions for Station #5. Dry mount copy on a manila file folder.

Directions for Station #5:

1. The rules for the Flame Game are beside the deck of cards.
2. The object of the game is to get rid of all of your cards and *not* have the FLAME Card at the end of the game.
3. Before your group starts to play, have one person read the directions for the game to everyone in the group.
4. When you finish the game, take one blank card. Think of a safety rule for "Walkers." Print the rule on the bottom of the card. Draw a picture of your own for the rule.
5. Put your card in the box on the table.
6. You are now ready to move to Station #6.

[5] Game developed by Marlyce Mizer and Linda Dubnicka, Kent State University, Kent, Ohio.

FLAME GAME CARDS

CARD	PICTURE	RULE
1.	Gasoline can	1. Store fluids properly.
2.	Matches in a pack	2. Don't play with matches.
3.	Fire alarm	3. Wait for help.
4.	Dial of a telephone	4. Know the fire department's phone number.
5.	A door	5. Close doors and windows.
6.	A window with a ladder	6. Don't jump. Use ladders.
7.	Diagram of a floor plan	7. Plan fire exits.
8.	Stick figures of a family-burning house in background	8. Get family to safety.
9.	A question mark	9. After reporting fire, wait for questions.
10.	A complete telephone	10. Call fire department.
11.	Electric cord plug	11. Don't overload sockets.
12.	Red Cross	12. First-aid for injuries.
13.	A flame	13. (no rule)

FLAME GAME DIRECTIONS

Any number of people can play this card game. Using all the cards in the deck, deal the cards around one at a time. If some players have one more card than others, it does not matter.

The object of the game is to get rid of your cards as quickly as possible by getting pairs, (example: two "Don't overload sockets," or two "Call fire departments"). Hold your cards fanshape. Remove any pairs (two of the same card) from your hand, read the safety rule out loud, and lay them face-down on the table. (If you have three of a kind, only two can be set down; if you have four of a kind, all four cards are set down because this makes two pairs.)

When all players have laid down all the pairs they hold, play begins; play moves to the player on the dealer's left.

The dealer takes any one card (he sees only the back of the card and does not know what he is getting) from the player on his left. If he can use the card to form a pair with one he holds, he reads the rule out loud and lays the pair face-down on the table. In this way he is ridding his hand of two cards, but he does not get another turn. If he does not match any card he holds, he must add the card he draws to those in his hand, hoping for better luck when his turn comes on the next round.

Everyone around the table takes a turn until finally all the cards have been paired and laid down except for the "Flame" card. The holder of this card is the FLAME. Remember, don't get caught holding the FLAME at the end of the game.

STATION #6: DESIGN YOUR OWN

Directions: (Teacher)

You have the idea for Station Learning. Design your own for this station.

---

concept 4:

The Potential for Hazards and Accidents Exists, Whatever the Environment.

Introduction to Concept — Upper Elementary Level

ACCIDENTS DON'T JUST HAPPEN

Accidents cause more young people your age to be hurt and even to die than anything else. What is an accident? What are some of the kinds of accidents that have happened to you or to someone you know in the past week? the past year? Could these accidents have been prevented? How?

Accidents don't just happen. They are *caused* by something a person either *does* or *fails to do*. Think about the accident you just told us about. Was it caused by something you *did*, or would something you *did not do* have prevented the accident from happening? Since all accidents are *caused* by people, and since no person is perfectly in control of his *thinking*, his *feelings*, and what he is *doing* all of the time, there will always be accidents. What we need to do is try to cut down on the number of accidents, especially serious accidents that could cause you or someone you know to be badly hurt — or even die.

In this concept you will be *learning* to recognize the kinds of accidents that can happen to you or those people around you, how they happen, and how they might be prevented from happening. You will be examining the *feelings* you have when you find yourself faced with a dangerous situation. In addition, you will be doing some activities to help remind you and others to "think safety" all of the time.

CONTINUOUS PROGRESS LEARNING

To the Teacher:

Another method of providing learning experiences that you may want to explore and utilize is Continuous Progress Learning (CPL). In this method you would prepare packets of learning activities with challenges for students based upon their levels of learning. It is suggested that packets be developed on three levels for (1) slow learners, (2) average learners, and (3) honors students.

In preparing these learning packets, it should be noted that the same general behavioral objective is used for all three levels, but the specific behavioral objectives used to attain the general objective will vary according to the learning experiences that are designed for the ability level. All learning experiences contained in the packets should be designed to be carried out by the student on an individual basis. No group learnings, skits, or class discussions would be appropriate.

CPL is valuable not only because of the consideration for ability levels, but also because the student may progress at his/her own pace, moving ahead through the concept as he/she is ready.

You must understand that CPL packets can only be developed over a period of time. It will take time and thoughtful planning for you to complete the packets for the health concept(s) you choose to use in your grade for the school year. For this reason, it may be prudent to establish a writing team of teachers in your grade either within your own school or from other schools to ease the burden. This way there can also be fresh ideas and creativity included because of the viewpoints of different teachers. Once completed, CPL may prove to be a very gratifying experience for both you and your students. In ensuing years you will need only to discard ineffectual parts of the packets, insert new ideas, revise those retained, and develop new packets in other concepts.

In this concept dealing with accident/safety education at the upper elementary level, an example of CPL is provided using one general behavioral objective on the three levels of learning. Perhaps this will increase your interest in trying to develop more learning packets in this concept or in another concept of your choice.

CPL: School Safety Campaign
(Slow Learner Packet)

Concept:

The potential for hazards and accidents exists, whatever the environment.

General Behavioral Objective:

The student will be able to identify ways of preventing physical injuries in a variety of environments.

Grade Level: Upper elementary

Directions: (Teacher)

1. CPL packets contain:
   a. An introduction that sets the stage for the learning experiences included in the packet.
   b. Directions for the series of learning experiences.
      1. Where to get any worksheets needed for the activity.
      2. Where to find any needed reference materials.
      3. Where to do the activity if a specialized area is needed.
      4. What to do with any product when finished.
2. All worksheets for the learning experiences are usually organized in a designated location.
3. A time limit is normally set for the completion of this phase of learning with a minimum level of accomplishment. For example: We will be using CPL packets for three weeks. There are five packets prepared for each color group. By the end of that time, you must have completed Blue Packet #1. If you finish before this time, work through as many of the other packets in your color as you have time to do and do well.

Introduction to Blue Packet #1:

All of the people assigned to this packet (PAK-ket) are members of the Pre-Teen Advertising (AD-vuhr-tie-zing) Company. Your company has been hired to develop (dee-VEL-up) a school safety campaign (kam-PANE) to make _____ school a safer place to be. Each activity in this packet is one part of your job.

You are trying to get the students in the school to become more aware of what each of them can do to prevent injuries to themselves and to others.

ACTIVITY #1

Domain: Cognitive   *Dimension:* Physical

Specific Behavioral Objective:

Given a list of school environments from which to choose, the student will be able to describe two ways to prevent physical injury by making a poster with a slogan.

Introduction:

You have been asked by your boss to make two posters to remind everyone of things they *should do* or *should not do* to keep from having an accident.

Each poster is to have a safety slogan (SLOW-gun). A slogan is a catchy phrase used in advertising to sell an idea, a product, or a service. Here are two examples of slogans:

Running in the hall may cause you to fall.

"Can" your trash.

You can think of others that are even better, so don't use these examples for your posters.

Directions:

1. Choose two different places in the school where accidents can happen.
2. Make up a safety slogan for each place and write both on a piece of scratch paper.
3. Check your spelling in the dictionary. If you have problems, ask the teacher for help.
4. Plan the colors you want to use to catch the eyes of the other students.
5. Get two pieces of poster paper from the supply table. Use one for each slogan.

6. Either draw a picture for each slogan or find a picture in the magazines on the table.

7. Print and color the slogans.

8. Put your name on the posters.

9. Give them to the teacher.

10. You are now ready to do Activity #2.

To the Teacher:

Activity #1 is developed. For the remainder of the activities in this packet, only ideas in the form of specific behavioral objectives are provided. In each case, the activities are related to the general behavioral objective stated previously. Try your hand at designing the rest of the packet.

ACTIVITY #2

Domain: Affective   *Dimension:* Physical

Specific Behavioral Objective:

The student will be able to explain the importance of improving safety practices at school by writing a spot announcement for the public address system.

ACTIVITY #3

Domain: Cognitive   *Dimension:* Physical

Specific Behavioral Objective:

When given a checklist, the student, by surveying the area, will be able to identify the existing conditions in one area of the school which could cause physical injuries.

ACTIVITY #4

Domain: Affective   *Dimension:* Physical

Specific Behavioral Objective:

Using the completed checklist, the student will be able to suggest a plan to repair or remove one of the identified hazards by describing the condition and the plan of action on a tape recording.

ACTIVITY #5

Domain: Psychomotor   *Dimension:* Physical

Specific Behavioral Objective:

With art supplies, the student will be able to make a collage of things used in the school which, if not used properly, could cause physical injury.

CPL: The Safety Expert
(Average Learner Packet)

Concept:

The potential for hazards and accidents exists, whatever the environment.

General Behavioral Objective:

The student will be able to describe ways of preventing physical injury in a variety of environments.

Grade Level: Upper elementary

Directions: (Teacher)

1. CPL packets contain:
   a. An introduction that sets the stage for the learning experiences included in the packet.
   b. Directions for each of the learning experiences.
   1. Where to get any worksheets needed for the activity.
   2. Where to find any needed reference materials.
   3. Where to do the activity if a specialized area is needed.
   4. What to do with any product when finished.
2. All worksheets for the learning experiences are usually organized in a designated location.
3. A time limit is normally set for the completion of this phase of learning with a minimum level of accomplishment. For example: We will be using CPL packets for three weeks. There are five packets prepared for each color group. By the end of that time, you must have completed Red Packet #1. If you finish before this time, work through as many of the other packets in your color as you have time to do and do well.

Introduction to Red Packet #1:

You are a world famous safety expert. At the present time, you have a radio program, a television program, a newspaper column, and you

126

also write articles for magazines. You think it is very important to help people lead safer lives.

Since you can't know everything there is to know about safety, you often have to use reference material to help you give correct information.

ACTIVITY #1

Domain: Cognitive   *Dimension:* Physical

Specific Behavioral Objective:

The student will be able to demonstrate a knowledge of ways to prevent physical injury by writing responses to a series of "Dear Safety Expert" letters.

Directions:

In your mail today are letters that must be answered for publication in your newspaper column.

1. Read each letter carefully.
2. The safety books and pamphlets to use for reference are on the cart in the back of the room.
3. Write an answer to each letter giving good safety advice to the letter writer.
4. Sign each letter with your own name.
5. Put the letters in the box under the *Red* sign.

LETTERS

Dear Safety Expert:

I have a very good friend. We enjoy doing lots of neat things together. Last night I slept at his house. While watching TV, I noticed that every electrical outlet in the room had four or five cords plugged in. My dad says that this is dangerous and I can't stay at his house all night any more. If my dad is right, what can I do? I'd hate to have anything happen to my buddy.

—Socket-to-em

Dear Safety Expert:

Everyday when we ride to school in the school bus, there is a group of four or five kids that horse around. Recently they have been throwing things that belong to other kids. The bus driver has tried to make them settle down, but she never seems to see them when they are at their worst. I am afraid something might hit the driver and cause an accident. Is there anything I can do without being a tattle-tale?

—No Rat Fink

Dear Safety Expert:

The other day, when my friend and I were walking to school, a stranger drove up in a car and asked us if we wanted a ride to school. We are old enough to know better so we said "No!" and ran away. Now I worry about the younger kids who walk. Perhaps the stranger will try again. I saw the person, and I know what kind of car the person was in. What do you think I should do?

—No Rides for Me

Dear Safety Expert:

I think I am old enough to stay in the house alone when my parents leave. They think that I still need a babysitter. What can I tell them to prove that I know how to stay safe and secure when they are not there?

—Not Afraid

Dear Safety Expert:

I have a big decision to make. My friends want me to go swimming in a deep quarry on the other side of town. I swim a little, but not very well. I like these kids and don't want to lose their friendship. I don't want to be called chicken but I am a little scared. Can you help me?

—Confused

Dear Safety Expert:

The other day, as we were watching TV, there was a tornado warning flashed on the screen. None of us knew what to do because we don't have a basement in our house. What should we do?

—Wants To Be Safe

Dear Safety Expert:

There is an old house in our neighborhood that is so rickety and wrecked it wouldn't take much for it to fall down. The windows are boarded up, and there are signs telling people to keep out, but some of the kids still play there. I'd like to tell people how dangerous this is, but I don't know how to go about it. What advice can you give me?

—Spooky

Dear Safety Expert:

Sometimes I have to babysit for my younger brother and sister. After Mom and Dad leave, I have trouble with them because they tell me I'm not their boss. I haven't said anything to anyone, but I'm scared that they will get hurt. They've made a game out of striking matches and blowing them out. I found them playing with Dad's gun, which none of us are to touch, and once they even locked me out of the house. What can I do?

—Worried Babysitter

To the Teacher:

Activity #1 is developed. For the remainder of the activities in this packet, only ideas in the form of specific behavioral objectives are provided. In each case, the activities are related to the general behavioral objective for the packet. Try your hand at designing the rest of the packet.

ACTIVITY #2

Domain: Psychomotor   *Dimension:* Physical

Specific Behavioral Objective:

Using one of the problems from the "Dear Safety Expert" letters, the student will be able to write and record an informative two-minute script about the dangers involved. (Radio Program)

ACTIVITY #3

Domain: Psychomotor   *Dimension:* Physical

Specific Behavioral Objective:

Using a selected problem from the "Dear Safety Expert" letters, the student will be able to make a poster that illustrates how to prevent the possible injury. (Television Program)

ACTIVITY #4

Domain: Affective   *Dimension:* Physical

Specific Behavioral Objective:

Drawing from any environment, the student will be able to develop five items he/she thinks should be included in a class booklet "Hints for Pre-Teen Safety."

CPL: Media Productions, Inc.
(Honors Learner Packet)

Concept:

The potential for hazards and accidents exists, whatever the environment.

General Behavioral Objective:

The student will be able to describe ways of preventing physical injury in a variety of environments.

Domain: Cognitive   *Dimension:* Physical

Grade Level: Upper elementary

Directions: (Teacher)

1. CPL packets contain:
   a. An introduction that sets the stage for the learning experiences included in the packet.
   b. Directions for each of the learning experiences.
      1. Where to get any worksheets needed for the activity.
      2. Where to find any needed reference materials.
      3. Where to do the activity if a specialized area is needed.
      4. What to do with any product when finished.
2. All worksheets for the learning experiences are usually organized in a designated location.
3. A time limit is normally set for the completion of this phase of learning with a minimum level of accomplishment. For example: We will be using CPL packets for three weeks. There are five packets prepared for each color group. By the end of that time, you must have completed Green Packet #1. If you finish before this time, work through as many of the other packets in your color as you have time to do and do well.

Note to Teacher:

Because the activities in Green Packet #1 are very time consuming, there are only two rather than the usual four or five in most learning packets.

Introduction to Green Packet #1:

All of the people assigned to this packet work for the Media Productions, Inc. The company has accepted a job to produce a variety of safety materials to be used by elementary school students. Since there is a large production staff in your company, you can choose what part of the safety materials you want to develop.

ACTIVITY #1

Domain: Cognitive   *Dimension:* Physical

Specific Behavioral Objective:

When given a variety of situations in several environments, the student will be able to describe ways of preventing accidents or injury in a selected locale by creating a mock filmstrip.

Directions:

1. Your job is to create a mock filmstrip.
2. Choose one of the activities from the following list. If there is one of particular interest to you that isn't on the list, have it approved by the teacher.

    a. cooking in the kitchen
    b. keeping safe and secure at home
    c. keeping safe and secure on the street
    d. riding a bike
    e. outdoor camping
    f. hearing a tornado warning broadcast
    g. swimming in the lake/pond/river/creek/ocean
    h. swimming in a pool
    i. using a power mower
    j. babysitting
    k. playing on the playground
    l. riding in the school bus
    m. sled riding
    n. playing in physical education class
    o. skiing on the slopes
    p. riding in a car
    q. horseback riding
    r. skating (board, roller, ice)
    s. storing medicines
    t. playing football

3. Using a piece of scratch paper, write out a list of safety rules to prevent accidents for your choice of activity. Reference materials are on the Resource table for your use.

4. Sketch a small picture that will illustrate each safety rule.

5. Count the number of pictures you will have in your film strip. These are called "frames." Add two extra frames to your number: one for a "title," one for "The End."

6. Measure the width of the screen in the box where you will show your filmstrip.

7. Roll out the shelf paper and measure off 4 inches for as many widths as you have frames, plus another 4 inches. Measure 4 inches, draw a vertical line. Then measure off the width for each frame and draw vertical lines to separate the frames. Be sure to have 4 inches left at the end. Cut strip off of roll.

8. On the first frame write or print your title.

9. Draw your pictures on the rest of the frames. On the last frame write or print "The End."

10. Make your pictures colorful and attractive by using crayons or watercolors.

ACTIVITY #2

Domain: Psychomotor   *Dimension:* Physical

Specific Behavioral Objective:

Using the illustrations on the mock filmstrips, the student will be able to write and record a script that will describe ways of preventing physical injuries.

Directions:

1. Write a script to go with your filmstrip.

2. Use this form for the script.

Frame #	*Script*
Title	_____
1	_____
2	_____
etc.	

3. Show your filmstrip and the script to your teacher.

4. When it is okayed, record it on a cassette.

5. Label the cassette with the title of your filmstrip and your name.

6. Glue one end of the film strip to the dowel between the marks on the dowel. The marks show the width of the screen.

7. Glue the other end of the filmstrip to the other dowel between the marks.

8. Wipe off any extra glue. When dry, roll filmstrip on the dowel closest to "The End" frame.

9. Put a rubber band around the filmstrip. Give filmstrip and cassette to your teacher.

---

concept 5:

There are Reciprocal Relationships Involving
Man, Disease and Environment.

Introduction to Concept — Lower Elementary Level

JEREMIAH THE TRAVELING GERM

Have you ever seen Jeremiah the Traveling Germ? He comes in many sizes and shapes, and he really gets around. Sometimes he travels by water, and other times he takes to the air to get where he wants to go. You may help him to get around by carrying him on your fingers. He especially likes to hang out under your fingernails with the hope that you will take him to your mouth.

Jeremiah is not a welcome visitor. He doesn't bring you toys or candy when he comes to see you. But in his bag he has many surprises that he *may* give to you. Perhaps there will be a stomach ache, a fever, chills, pain, coughing, sneezing, or even red bumps on your

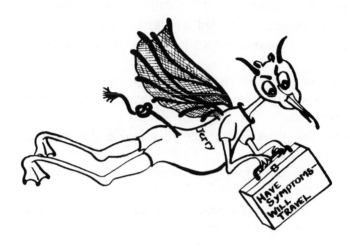

skin — all of the nasty things you really don't want. After a while he may get tired of visiting you and leave to start traveling again to take his gifts somewhere else.

You may never see Jeremiah the Traveling Germ — but he is looking for you!

The Jeremiah Germ Game[6]

Concept:

There are reciprocal relationships involving man, disease, and environment.

General Behavioral Objective:

The student will be able to describe ways of keeping healthy.

Domain: Cognitive   *Dimension:* Mental

Grade Level: Lower elementary

---

[6] Developed by Mary Elaine Seidenwand, School of Public Health, University of Michigan, Ann Arbor, Michigan.

Specific Behavioral Objective:

The student will be able to read ways to protect people from communicable diseases by playing the "Jeremiah Germ" game.

Directions: (Teachers)

1. Prepare the "Jeremiah Germ" gameboard (see p. 137) and the Chance Cards (see p. 136). It is suggested that the game materials be produced on tagboard and laminated.
2. Duplicate rules for the game (see p. 135).
3. Game may be used at a Learning Station or during free time.

JEREMIAH GERM GAME RULES

1. Read the rules aloud to all players.
2. Two to four players.
3. Each player selects a playing piece and places it on "START."
4. Place CHANCE cards face down on the area marked "CHANCE."
5. Each player rolls the die. Player with highest number begins first with others taking turns in clockwise direction.
6. Playing piece is moved the number of spaces indicated on the die. Player then reads the message and follows any directions given.
7. When a player lands on "CHANCE," a card is taken from the CHANCE card deck, read aloud, directions followed, and the card is returned to the bottom of the deck.
8. Any player landing in "Jeremiah's Germ Jail" must roll a "2" or a "4" to be released from jail. If either number is rolled, the player stays in jail until his *next* turn, at which time he moves the number of spaces indicated by the roll of the die on that turn.
9. The player who reaches the "HEALTH HOUSE" first is the winner.
10. In order to enter the "HEALTH HOUSE," a player must roll the exact number that is needed to cover the spaces.
11. No player may roll the die twice in succession unless the chance card is drawn that says "Take Another Turn."

CHANCE CARDS

Directions:

Make chance cards in contrasting color to the board to fit the space provided for them on the game board. Put the message on one side of the card and the words CHANCE CARD on the other.

BROKE A BLISTER	KILLED A FLY!
Go back 1 Space	Move Ahead 1 Space

STAYED HOME WHEN SICK	KEPT FOOD COVERED
Go Ahead 1 Space	Take Another Turn

YOU PICKED YOUR NOSE	YOU BITE YOUR FINGERNAILS
Skip Next Turn	Go Back 1 Space

WASHED FRUIT BEFORE EATING	USED YOUR OWN DRINKING GLASS
Go Ahead 2 Spaces	Go to Free Space

LICKED ANOTHER'S ICE CREAM CONE	ATE CANDY THAT FELL ON GROUND
Skip Next Turn	Go To Jail

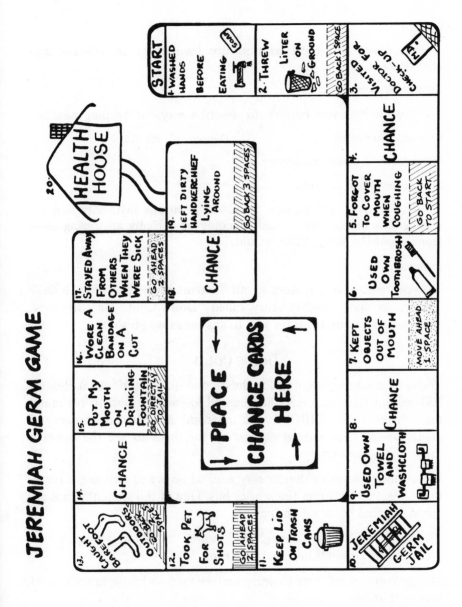

JEREMIAH GERM GAME

Don's Cold[7]

Concept:

There are reciprocal relationships involving man, disease, and environment.

General Behavioral Objective:

The student will be able to describe ways of keeping healthy.

Domain: Cognitive   *Dimension:* Mental

Grade Level: Lower elementary

Specific Behavioral Objective:

The student will be able to identify various behaviors that encourage/discourage the spread of colds by verbally answering questions about the story, "Don's Cold."

Introduction:

Do you remember the story about "Jeremiah the Traveling Germ"? Today, we have another story called "Don's Cold." In this story, there are some questions for you to answer as we go along.

DON'S COLD

Today was an unusual day for the second grade students at Beacon Hill School. It was a day they had all looked forward to for many many weeks—the CIRCUS was in town! Mr. Nelson, the second grade teacher, had special permission for them to see the opening show that afternoon.

It was about noon as the 26 very excited boys and girls began forming a line and boarding the school bus. One of the students, though, could not find his usual bus partner.

"Where is Don?" Jerry thought to himself. "Surely he wouldn't miss school today. Something *must* be wrong."

Mr. Nelson walked over to Jerry and seemed to know exactly what he was thinking.

---

[7] Developed by Mary Elaine Seidenwand, School of Public Health, University of Michigan, Ann Arbor, Michigan.

"Jerry," Mr. Nelson said, "I'm afraid Don won't be going with us to the circus today. His mother called the school office early this morning and said he has a very bad cold. No lion tamers for him — only a 'germ-tamer' — his doctor!"

Feeling very disappointed, Jerry climbed the steps onto the school-bus and sank into an empty seat. As the bus left the school grounds and started on its way, Jerry just stared out the window. He didn't feel much like talking or joking with his classmates. All he could think about was the big show they had talked about for weeks and how Don would miss it.

"Why did Don have to get sick today of *all* days?" Jerry thought. "He was fine on Friday. Jeremiah Germ must have chosen Don as his latest victim! But why," Jerry wondered, "did Don get sick while I'm feeling fine? The two of us do almost all of the same things, so why don't I have a fever and cold too?"

Jerry thought about his last question very carefully. He remembered they had walked home from school together last Friday. It was rainy and cool outside, but Don was not dressed for the weather. Instead he wore only a sweater. Jerry, though, was dressed correctly. . . .

(To Students):

    1. What kind of clothing do you think Jerry was wearing?

"Don *did* seem to be shivering," Jerry recalled.

Next his mind shifted to those things they talked about on the way home. Don said that all he does after school or on weekends is stay inside and watch TV. He's even seen all the reruns of his favorite shows. Jerry replied that he watches a few cartoons on Saturday mornings, but spends most of his free time outdoors. . . .

(To Students):

    1. Name some things you think Jerry does on weekends or after school.

    2. How do these activities help Jerry stay healthy?

Jerry then mentioned to Don the appointment he'd had with his family doctor.

Don just laughed. "I haven't been to the doctor or dentist in years!" he said. "Why bother going if you aren't sick?". . .

(To Students):

   1. Who will volunteer to be Jerry?

   2. Explain to us why visits to the doctor are necessary even when you're not sick.

   3. How many of you go to the doctor for check-ups when you're not sick?

Jerry also remembered Don bragged about staying up late each evening — almost until the end of the news broadcasts — even when there was school the following day. And Don's babysitter let *him choose* his own bedtime.

"I'm lucky," Don said. "I don't need much sleep.". . .

(To Students):

   1. Do you think Don is lucky being able to stay up so late?

Jerry doesn't consider himself lucky or unlucky, just smart. He knows he needs a good night's sleep every day. . . .

(To Students):

   1. Why does Jerry need a good night's sleep?

The two boys soon reached Don's place.

"Come in and rest awhile before walking the rest of the way to your house," said Don. "Maybe the rain will let up by then." It sounded like a good idea to Jerry and so they both went inside.

"How about something to eat?" Don asked. "I'm having my usual — a candy bar and a bottle of pop. Want the same?" Jerry looked at the clock and knew that he'd be eating supper in another hour. All those sweets would ruin his appetite, not to mention what they'd do for his teeth; the dentist had warned him last time! So instead Jerry had a snack which was much better for him. . . .

(To Students):

   1. What kind of snack might Jerry have had?

   2. What kind of snacks do you have after school?

When Jerry stopped to put all of these thoughts together — not dressing for the weather, lack of exercise and fresh air, not visiting the doctor regularly, not getting much sleep, and eating junk foods —

Jerry realized why Don was sick and he himself was healthy. Yes, the two of them were alike in many ways—both played baseball, liked crossword puzzles, wrote poetry, and loved peanut butter-and-banana sandwiches. But Jerry knew what was and wasn't good for him and took better care of himself. Jeremiah the Traveling Germ never had much of a chance to work on him.

"Hmmm. . . ." exclaimed Jerry. "Maybe Don doesn't know about this germ thing, but I'm sure he'd be happy to learn! When he's feeling better, I'll tell him the story about Jeremiah. And maybe next year we'll both see the circus—together!"

Suggested Follow-Up:

Discussion:

1. What health behaviors can help us prevent illness?
2. Which behaviors do you practice?
3. Which behaviors do you not practice?

I Spy[8]

Concept:

There are reciprocal relationships involving man, disease, and environment.

General Behavioral Objective:

The student will be able to identify various forms of environmental pollutants.

Domain: Psychomotor   *Dimension:* Social

Grade Level: Lower elementary

Specific Behavioral Objective:

The student will be able to demonstrate a sense of responsibility for the environment by helping to remove litter from the school grounds.

---

[8] Developed by Mary Elaine Seidenwand, School of Public Health, University of Michigan, Ann Arbor, Michigan.

Directions: (Teacher)

1. Mark five plastic trash bags with a felt tip marker "Sad Scrap Sack."
2. Select a detective from the class.
3. Explain the rules for "I Spy."
4. Practice game in classroom.
5. Divide class into groups of five or six each with a detective.
6. Assign each group to a specific area of the school grounds.

Directions: (Student)

1. One person is the detective.
2. The detective sees a piece of litter within the specific boundaries.
3. The detective says, "I spy," and describes the object to the other players.
4. Each player has a turn to guess the object.
5. When a player correctly identifies the object, the *detective* picks up the object and puts it in the group's "Sad Scrap Bag."
6. The player correctly naming the object becomes the next detective and the game continues.

Suggested Follow-Up:

1. Identify the types of litter found in each area.
2. Weigh the trash picked up by the class.
3. Discuss what each person can do to keep the classroom, the school and the school ground free from litter.

There are Reciprocal Relationships Involving
Man, Disease, and Environment.

Introduction to Concept — Upper Elementary

THE WISHBONE

"Dinner is ready!" announced Grandma.

It didn't take another word to get everyone scrambling to their feet
and seated at the huge table heavy with steaming food. After everyone was settled and the thanks were given, Grandma ushered in the
largest turkey Jamie had ever seen and set it in front of Grandpa to
be carved.

Jamie loved Thanksgiving, not only because of the food, but also
because it was a time when all of the family gathered together to
share their happiness.

Grandpa was an expert in carving the turkey. It wasn't long until
only the bones were showing. He stopped for a moment from his
chore and proudly proclaimed that he had found the wishbone.
When everyone had quieted down, he said that he was going to give
the wishbone to Jamie and Jimmy because they were the youngest
members of the family — but only if the one who had the largest
piece of the bone after breaking it would share his/her wish with the
family. Jamie and Jimmy quickly agreed.

After the bone snapped, Jamie was surprised to see that she was
holding the larger piece. It was up to her to make the wish and
announce it to the family. She could think of so many wonderful
things she wished for.

Jamie looked around at all of the happy faces and quickly said, "I've
got it! I know what I will wish for!"

What do you suppose Jamie would wish for?

"My wish," said Jamie, "is that everyone in this room will always be healthy so that we can spend every Thanksgiving together, just as we are."

Do you think that only wishing to be healthy and free from disease will make it so?

Why?

What do you think you, and all others, can do to prevent illness?

Who Knows About A Zoonose?[9]

Concept:

There are reciprocal relationships involving man, disease, and environment.

General Behavioral Objective:

The student will be able to demonstrate an understanding about zoonoses.

Domain: Cognitive   *Dimension:* Physical

Grade Level: Upper elementary

Specific Behavioral Objective:

After an explanation of zoonoses, the student will be able to identify preventative measures to be taken by verbally listing.

Directions: (Teacher)

1. Zoonoses are animal diseases that are transmitted from animals to man.
2. Adapt this lesson to the animals in your environment — e.g., rats/bubonic plague; wild rabbits/tularemia — and so on.
3. This lesson deals with zoonoses that occur in three common household pets: dogs, cats, and birds.
4. Make transparencies of: Doggie Do's and Don'ts, p. 146; Cat Cans and Cannots, p. 146; and Parrot - Pleasers and Punishers, p. 147.

Introduction:

Have you ever caught a cold from a family member or friend?

[9] Developed by Dawn Hilston, Allied Health Sciences Department, Kent State University, Kent, Ohio.

Did you know that you can catch some diseases from your pets too? Well, you can! These diseases are called zoonoses. (Write word on chalkboard and have students pronounce it.)

Today we're going to learn about three different zoonoses. The first zoonose is rabies.

Do you know what rabies is? Yes, it's also called hydrophobia, and it's a disease caused by a virus that infects animals. People can also get rabies if they are bitten by an animal that has the disease.

From which animals do you know you could get rabies (a bat, a fox, a wolf, dog, cat, skunk)? The most common animal that you can get rabies from is a dog.

How many of you have a dog? What do your parents do to protect your dog and your family from getting rabies?

Yes, they take the dog to the veterinarian every ___ years (check on the requirement in your state for rabies immunization) for a shot that will protect your dog from getting rabies.

What are some of the things we can do to prevent rabies? (List answers.)

Another zoonose is Cat Scratch Fever. Cat Scratch Fever is a disease you can get from a scratch or bite from an infected cat.

How can we avoid Cat Scratch Fever? (List answers.)

The third zoonose is Parrot Fever (Psittacosis). You can get this disease from any infected bird (parakeet, pigeon, poultry). With this disease, the bird doesn't have to bite you. The virus can be in the bird droppings or on the feathers. How can we avoid this zoonose? (List answers.)

Suggested Follow-Up:

1. Verbally review the preventative measures for each disease.
   a. Rabies — Do's and Don'ts
   b. Cat Scratch Fever — Do's and Don'ts
   c. Psittacosis — Do's and Don'ts
2. Show transparencies
3. Choose one of the pets and write a story on "Having Fun with My
   _____." The story is to include one positive and one negative measure to prevent contracting the zoonose.

Doggie Do's and Don'ts.

Do:

1. GET YOUR DOG A LICENSE.

2. KEEP YOUR DOG TIED UP.

3. TAKE YOUR DOG TO THE VET FOR RABIES SHOT.

Don't:

1. PET STRAY DOG'S.

2. TEASE YOUR DOG.

Cat Cans and Cannots

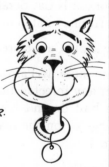

CANS:

1. WASH ANY SCRATCH OR BITE WITH SOAP AND WATER. TELL AN ADULT ABOUT THE SCRATCH OR BITE.

2. WASH HANDS AFTER CHANGING KITTY LITTER.

CANNOTS:

1. PICK ON THE CAT OR IT MIGHT PICK ON YOU.

2. DISTURB THE CAT WHILE HE IS EATING.

PARROT PLEASERS
AND PUNISHERS

PLEASERS:
1. WASH HANDS AFTER
CLEANING BIRD CAGE.

2. TAKE A SICK BIRD
TO THE VET.

PUNISHERS:
1 GO NEAR A SICK BIRD.

2. RUB YOUR EYES OR PUT YOUR
FINGERS IN YOUR MOUTH WHEN
PLAYING WITH THE BIRD.

Afraid — Who, Me?[10]

Concept:

There are reciprocal relationships involving man, disease and environment.

General Behavioral Objective:

The student will be able to explain the value of preventing diseases.

Domain: Affective   *Dimension:* Emotional

Grade Level: Upper elementary

Specific Behavioral Objective:

Given a series of preventative actions, the student will be able to identify the degree of fear each produces by placing them on a forced choice ladder diagram.

[10] Developed by Dawn Hilston, Allied Health Sciences, Kent State University, Kent, Ohio.

Directions: (Teacher)

1. Reproduce and distribute copies of the forced choice ladder diagram (see page 149).
2. Read Directions for "Afraid—Who, Me?" to students.
3. Read each action and give time to write letter on rung.
4. After all 10 actions are read, repeat and give two minutes to rearrange choices. Answers can be crossed out, erased, or arrows drawn to new rungs.

Suggested Follow-Up:

1. Discussion of why we fear things.
   a. Fear of the unknown is natural.
   b. Some procedures are unpleasant or hurt, but if the actions aren't taken the consequences are more unpleasant.
2. Tabulate the actions that are "most feared" (Rungs #9 and 10) and those that are "least feared" (Rungs #1 and 2).
3. Discuss:
   a. Why individuals selected actions on Rungs #9 and 10.
   b. Why individuals selected actions on Rungs #1 and 2.
   c. What the consequences could be if the actions "most feared" were refused.

AFRAID—WHO, ME?

Directions:

1. Below Rung #1 of the ladder, write "Least Feared."
2. Above Rung #10 write "Most Feared."
3. Each of the actions that are listed help physicians or dentists prevent, diagnose, or cure disease.
4. As each action is read, put the *LETTER* of the action on the rung of the ladder according to how much or how little you fear having that done to you.
5. What you put on Rung #1 is feared very little or not at all; what you fear the most in being cared for when ill or injured is put on Rung #10.
6. Remember, there are no correct or incorrect answers. Put the letters on the ladder according to how much *you* fear the action.
7. After all of the actions have been read, you'll have two minutes to change your answers.

Actions:

    A. Having x-rays

    B. Having bands (braces) put on the teeth

    C. Having an operation

    D. Staying overnight in the hospital for observation

    E. Swallowing pills or other medicines

    F. Having blood taken from a finger or an arm

    G. Having the physician listen to your heart and lungs

    H. Having stitches put in a cut

    I . Getting a shot in the arm or in the hip

    J . Having a cavity filled

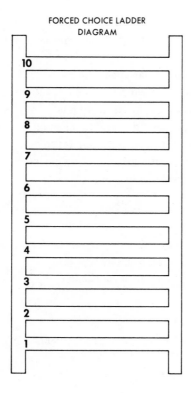

FORCED CHOICE LADDER
DIAGRAM

Stop Cardiovascular Disease[11]

Concept:

There are reciprocal relationships involving man, disease, and environment.

General Behavioral Objective:

The student will be able to identify the leading causes of death in the United States.

Domain: Psychomotor   *Dimension:* Mental

Grade Level: Upper elementary

Specific Behavioral Objective:

After completing the fill-in sentences, the student will be able to use the preventions for cardiovascular disease to draw the correct pathway through a maze.

Directions: (Teacher)

    1. Introduce word "Cardiovascular."

    2. Reproduce and distribute "Stop Cardiovascular Disease" (see p. 152).

    3. Key for fill-in sentences:

       Preventing Cardiovascular disease means:

       a. To have a thorough medical (*check-up*) each year.

       b. To avoid foods (*high*) in saturated fats.

       c. To eat a well-balanced diet and to maintain a desirable (*weight*).

       d. To get plenty of rest, fresh air, and (*exercise*).

       e. To refrain from starting the (*smoking*) habit.

       f. To reduce (*worry*) and tension.

Suggested Follow-Up:

    1. Discussion:

       a. Purpose and functions of the American Heart Association.

       b. Location of the local chapter.

       c. Services provided by the local chapter.

[11] Developed by Mary Elaine Seidenwand, School of Public Health, University of Michigan, Ann Arbor, Michigan.

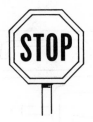

STOP CARDIOVASCULAR DISEASE

Directions:

a. Complete the following sentences by supplying the missing words.

b. Find your way through the maze below. The fill-in words will help act as guides. Good luck!

Preventing Cardiovascular Disease Means:

1. To have a thorough medical _____ each year.
2. To avoid foods _____ in saturated fats.
3. To eat a well-balanced diet and to maintain a desirable _____.
4. To get plenty of rest, fresh air, and _____.
5. To refrain from starting the _____ habit.
6. To reduce _____ and tension.

How Germs Come and Go[12]

Concept:

There are reciprocal relationships involving man, disease, and environment.

General Behavioral Objective:

The student will be able to discriminate between communicable and chronic illnesses.

[12] Developed by Mary Elaine Seidenwand, School of Public Health, University of Michigan, Ann Arbor, Michigan.

CARDIOVASCULAR DISEASE

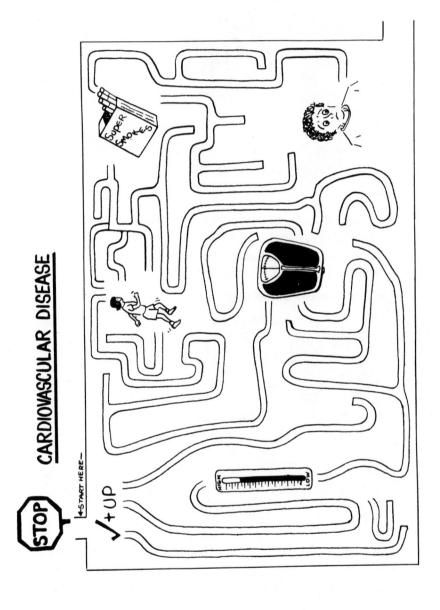

Domain: Cognitive   *Dimension:* Mental

Grade Level: Upper elementary

Specific Behavioral Objective:

With two teams playing Human Tic-Tac-Toe, the student will be able to identify the ways germs are communicated by responding to a series of questions.

Directions: (Teacher)

1. Make 8 inch "X's" out of construction paper for one-half of the class.
2. Make 8 inch "O's" for the other half of the class.
3. Punch two holes in the top of each letter. Tie a piece of string to each hole. String should be long enough to slip over students' heads.
4. Copy questions on separate index cards. Put answer on reverse side of each card.
5. Using six foot plastic tape strips, make a Tic-Tac-Toe game board on a 6' × 6' piece of heavy plastic. Each square will be 2' × 2'.
6. Designate a Master of Ceremonies to read the game questions and a scorekeeper.
7. Divide the rest of the class into two teams.
8. Each team forms a single file on opposite sides of the gameboard.
9. On the chalkboard, write:
   How Germs Come and Go:
   a. Contact/air
   b. Animals/insects
   c. Food/water

Suggested Follow-Up:

1. Discussion:
   a. Diseases missed twice during the game.
   b. Identify diseases common to the United States and those common to other parts of the world.

How Germs Come and Go

(HUMAN TIC-TAC-TOE)

Directions:

1. Object of the game is to get three of your team members standing on the gameboard in a vertical, horizontal, or diagonal line.

2. A coin is tossed to determine the starting team.

3. The Master of Ceremonies reads the first question to the first person on the starting team. If the question is answered correctly, the player stands in one of the unoccupied squares.

4. If the answer is incorrect, the player goes to the end of the file and the first person on the opposing team may answer the same question.

5. Any question missed twice is placed in a separate pile for discussion after the game is completed.

6. *No player may receive help from other members of the team, either in answering the question or in choosing the square in which to stand.*

7. Answers to all questions in this game are either "A," "B," or "C."

8. The scorekeeper gives one tally mark to the winning team. Three games are played. The team winning 2 out of 3 games is the Human Tic-Tac-Toe set winner.

9. Any game ending in a "draw" results in *both* teams receiving a tally mark.

Key:

How Germs Come and Go

    A. Contact/air
    B. Animals/Insects
    C. Food/water

Questions	*Answers*
1. Chicken Pox	A. Contact/air
2. Malaria	B. Animals/Insects
3. Cold	A. Contact/air
4. Botulism	C. Food/water
5. Flu	A. Contact/air
6. Polio	A. Contact/air
7. Rabies	B. Animals/Insects
8. Athlete's Foot	A. Contact/air
9. German Measles	A. Contact/air
10. Cholera	C. Food/water
11. Bubonic Plague	B. Animals/Insects
12. Smallpox	A. Contact/air

13. Dysentery	C. Food/water
14. Pneumonia	A. Contact/air
15. Yellow Fever	B. Animals/Insects
16. Meningitis	A. Contact/air
17. Mumps	A. Contact/air
18. Tetanus	A. Contact/air
19. Typhoid Fever	C. Food/water
20. Impetigo	A. Contact/air

concept 6:

The Family Serves to Perpetuate Man and Fulfill Certain Health Needs.

Introduction to Concept — Lower Elementary Level

THE CARDINAL FAMILY

Teacher Preparation:

Make mock birth announcements similar to the example and hand out to each pupil at the onset of the learning.

C. C. Cardinal and his beautiful mate, B. B., had been working very hard getting ready for the big day. They had searched the countryside for tiny twigs, pieces of string, small grass, grapevine, and anything else they could find to use in building their nest in the thick bushes on the edge of the woods. Their strong wings carried them back and forth hundreds of times until they were sure that they would have the best possible home for the babies that were on their way. The soft grasses and rootlets that lined the nest made it very comfortable.

One night as B. B. was settled in the nest, she laid three pale blue speckled eggs. B. B. and C. C. were excited because they knew that the eggs would hatch within the next two weeks. But they also knew

Birth Announcement

MR. AND MRS. C.C. CARDINAL
PROUDLY ANNOUNCE THE BIRTH OF
TRIPLETS ON MONDAY, MAY 2.
THE TRIPLETS EACH WEIGHED 10 GRAMS.

NAMES:
    C. C. CARDINAL JR.
    CAROL CARDINAL
    CAPPY CARDINAL

that they would have to keep the eggs warm and safe. Both took turns sitting in the nest.

C. C., Jr. was the first baby to hatch, followed closely by Carol and Cappy. Each was hungry immediately, so C. C. and B. B. went out to search for berries and seeds and insects to help the babies to grow strong. Cardinals take good care of their young before and after they are born.

What other ways, besides feeding, do you think C. C. and B. B. took care of their babies?

What can you tell the class about how dogs take care of their puppies after they are born?

What did your mother do for you while you were growing in her uterus? How did your father help get ready for your birth?

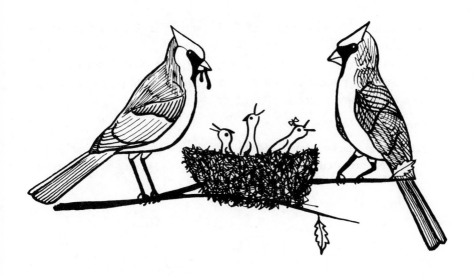

Parents Care!

Concept:

The family serves to perpetuate man and fulfill certain health needs.

General Behavioral Objective:

The student will be able to cite examples of how families fulfill the health needs of its members.

Domain: Psychomotor   *Dimension:* Physical

Grade Level: Lower elementary

Specific Behavioral Objective:

After hearing the Cardinal Family story, the student will be able to demonstrate one way that cardinals care for the physical needs of their young and one way that human parents care for theirs by drawing pictures.

Directions: (Student)

1. Fold your piece of drawing paper in half.

2. On one half of your paper, using your crayons, draw a

picture showing one way C. C. and B. B. Cardinal cared for
their babies.

3. On the other half of your paper, draw a picture showing one
   way your parents took care of your physical needs when you
   were a newborn baby.

Suggested Follow-Up:

1. Prepare a bulletin board with the title, *We Care for Our Children.*
2. After each student tells about his/her picture, tack the picture on the
   bulletin board.

My Needs Balloon

Concept:

The family serves to perpetuate man and fulfill certain health
needs.

General Behavioral Objective:

The student will be able to cite examples of how families fulfill
the health needs of its members.

Domain: Cognitive   *Dimension:* All

Grade Level: Lower elementary

Specific Behavioral Objective:

On a self-made balloon with a word or picture, the student will
be able to cite one way the family is providing for his/her physical,
mental-emotional or social health needs now.

Introduction:

The word NEED means something we must have. A HEALTH
NEED is something we must have to make our body work the way it
should, to make us happy, or to help us get along well with others.

Directions: (Student)

1. Take a piece of construction paper from the table. Choose
   any color you wish to make a pretend balloon.
2. With scissors, cut out the largest balloon you can from your
   colored paper.

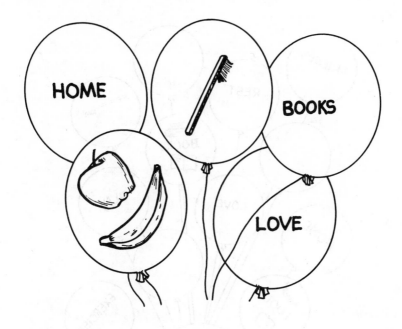

3. On your balloon you may either:

   a. Print a word that tells one way your family helps you to be healthy or happy, or

   b. Draw a picture of something that shows a health need your family contributes to you, or

   c. Cut out and paste on your balloon a picture from a magazine showing a health need your family provides for you.

4. When you finish, go to the table and take a piece of string. Paste your string to the bottom of your balloon.

Note to Teacher:

Make a large circle labeled "Me" and place it at the bottom of the bulletin board. Have students tack their balloons above and attach strings to the "Me" circle.

   1. Which balloons show things that make our bodies work well (physical needs)?

   2. Which balloons show things that make us happy (emotional needs)?

   3. Which balloons show things that help us get along well with others (social needs)?

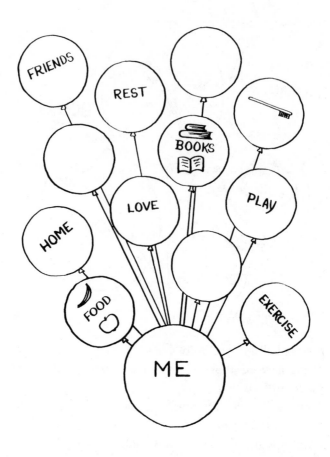

I Help My Family

Concept:

The family serves to perpetuate man and fulfill certain health needs.

General Behavioral Objective:

The student will be able to cite examples of how families fulfill the health needs of its members.

Domain: Affective   *Dimension:* All

Grade Level: Lower elementary

Specific Behavioral Objective:

The student will be able to suggest ways of helping to fulfill the physical, mental-emotional, or social health needs of the other family members by verbally completing stem sentences.

Introduction:

Each of you is a member of a family because none of you lives alone. You have seen the many ways your family has helped you to be healthy and happy. Now we will try to discover ways that *you* can help the other members of your family to be healthy and happy.

Directions:

I will read to you a part of a sentence. Tell me how you would finish that sentence.

1. I can help to make my home a safer place for everyone by . . .
2. I can show love for my family by . . .
3. I can help everyone in my family have more fun together by . . .
4. If I take good care of myself, it will help everyone in my family because . . .
5. I can set a good example for my family by . . .

Suggested Follow-Up:

Have students choose one way they believe they can best help their family. Each will take a turn acting out that behavior (as in charades). The student correctly guessing what the behavior is then gets to demonstrate the behavior he/she has chosen.

The Happy Home Family Catalogue[13]

Concept:

The family serves to perpetuate man and fulfill certain health needs.

[13] Developed by Dawn Hilston, Allied Health Sciences Department, Kent State University, Kent, Ohio.

General Behavioral Objective:

The student will be able to cite examples of how family members help fulfill the health needs of its members.

Domain: Affective   *Dimension:* All

Grade Level: Lower elementary

Specific Behavioral Objective:

Individually, the student will be able to describe the ways different members of a family contribute to the physical, emotional, or social well-being of the family by preparing a written description for a "Family Catalogue."

Introduction:

Have you ever seen a mail order catalogue?

What kind of things are described in these catalogues?

We're going to make a catalogue of our own today. Instead of describing clothes, toys, or things to use around the house, our catalogue will describe family members.

Did you ever wish you had a grandmother, a father, a brother, a sister, or a cousin like some of your friends? You know, not all of us have all of these relatives.

Our catalogue will have sections for grandparents, parents, brothers and sisters, aunts and uncles, and cousins.

Think about the relatives you have who help you meet your physical, emotional, or social needs. Think about the type of relative you wish you had who could help you meet your needs.

Now, you have some choices to make.

Directions: (Student)

1. Choose at least two relatives. They can be either real relatives or relatives you wish you had.
2. Write a description of each relative. The description should include what the person does or can do for your *physical, emotional,* or *social* health needs.

3. Use this as an example:

Title: Grandfather   #21

Description: Kind and jolly

Physical: Protects me by teaching me to swim.

Emotional: Makes me feel important by letting me help him make repairs around the house.

Social: Invites other kids to come and play with me when I visit his house.

Suggested Follow-Up:

1. Small group discussion:
   a. Share written descriptions.
   b. Discuss qualities liked in family member.
2. Class discussion:
   a. "What Kind of a Family Member Am I?"

---

concept 6:

The Family Serves to Perpetuate Man and Fulfill Certain Health Needs

---

Introduction to Concept — Upper Elementary Level

LINDA LITTLEFOX

Linda Littlefox was dashing swiftly through the woods and over the meadow towards her den. Her brothers and sisters were trying to keep up with her, but Linda had always been able to run faster than most of the other young foxes, and this made her a leader with them. She and her brothers and sisters and their many cousins had spent a busy afternoon playing. Now the sun was setting and Linda was feeling very hungry. Dinner would taste very good tonight! She wondered what her father and mother had found when they went hunting that morning. She thought to herself, "How much fun it is to run and play and then come home to the warmth and comfort of the Littlefox den with mother and father waiting. They must love each of us very much. They take such good care of us!''

Linda looked forward to the time when she would be able to have a family of her own. She would be such a good mother to her children! She would teach them to run and play, and when danger was near she would protect them. And if she found some little foxes who didn't have a mother or father, she would take them into her den and take care of them as if they were her own. She remembered her cousins whose mother and father went hunting one morning and never came home. Her mother took them into the happy Littlefox family and everyone loved them very much.

Now, as she was nearing the Littlefox den, Linda's sharp sense caught the welcome odor of food. She knew dinner was ready. "Aren't families wonderful?'' she thought to herself.

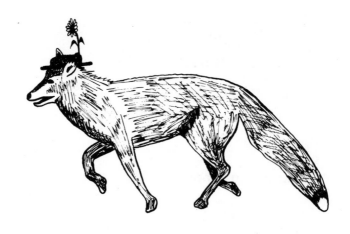

Family Mobile[14]

Concept:

The family serves to perpetuate man and fulfill certain health needs.

[14] Developed by Dawn Hilston, Allied Health Sciences Department, Kent State University, Kent, Ohio.

General Behavioral Objective:

The student will be able to describe the personal characteristics influenced by heredity.

Domain: Cognitive   *Dimension:* Physical

Grade Level: Upper elementary

Specific Behavioral Objective:

After a lecturette about heredity, the student will be able to identify inherited characteristics by making a mobile.

Directions: (Teacher)

1. Prepare lecturette on inherited and acquired characteristics.
2. Arrange for materials needed for mobile: coat hangers, string, white construction paper, colored pencils, crayons, or water paint.

Directions: (Student)

1. Construct a mobile of the members of your family.
2. Make (trace, if necessary) human figure forms for family members on white construction paper.
3. Add physical characteristics: color of eyes, hair, skin; curly or straight hair; facial features.
4. Tie string to hole in head and mobile. Adjust for balance.

Suggested Follow-Up:

1. Display mobiles.
2. Discussion of:
   a. What characteristics students inherited.
   b. What characteristics students have acquired.

Agree or Disagree[15]

Concept:

The family serves to perpetuate man and fulfill certain health needs.

---

[15] Developed by Mary Elaine Seidenwand, School of Public Health, University of Michigan, Ann Arbor, Michigan.

General Behavioral Objective:

The student will be able to identify the various male-female roles.

Domain: Affective   *Dimension:* Social

Grade Level: Upper elementary

Specific Behavioral Objective:

Using a computer program, the student will be able to express an opinion about male-female roles by responding to a series of statements involving family responsibilities.

Directions: (Teacher)

    1. Have the lesson programmed for the school computer.

    2. If computer terminals are not available, duplicate the questions.

Directions: (Student)

Type the letter of the response which describes you best.
Information:

1. I am	a. Female
	b. Male
2. I live with	a. Father only
	b. Mother only
	c. Both father and mother
	d. Other relative
	e. None of the above
3. I have	a. 0 sisters
	b. 1-2 sisters
	c. 3-4 sisters
	d. 5 or more sisters
4. I have	a. 0 brothers
	b. 1-2 brothers
	c. 3-4 brothers
	d. 5 or more brothers
5. I am	a. The only child in the family
	b. The youngest child in the family
	c. The oldest child in the family
	d. A middle child in the family

Directions:

There are NO correct answers to the following statements. Type the letter which tells how much you agree or disagree with the statement.

A. Strongly Agree
B. Agree
C. Disagree
D. Strongly Disagree

1. The father should be the head of the household.
2. Mothers should work only if the family needs the money to get along.
3. Both parents should share the job of disciplining the children.
4. Housework should be done only by the females in the family.
5. Housework should be shared by both males and females in the family.
6. It's just as important for boys to learn to cook as for girls.
7. Shopping for groceries is just as much a man's job as a woman's.
8. When important matters are being decided, all members of the family should be asked to give their opinions.
9. Females are better than males in managing the family finances.
10. Whoever is better at managing the family finances should do so.
11. The sex of a person should not determine who does a particular job around the house.
12. When a household chore needs to be done, the person with the time or the ability to do the job should do it.
13. Only men or boys should mow the lawn.
14. Only women or girls should cook and clean.
15. Mothers are more understanding than fathers.
16. Fathers are more understanding than mothers.
17. When their baby cries during the night, the mother and father should take turns getting up to care for the child.

18. Chores of family members should be rotated from week to week.

19. If the mother works, the father and children should prepare the meals.

20. If both parents work, both should share the household chores.

21. If both parents work, it's not fair to expect the mother to prepare all of the meals and clean the house.

22. When both parents work, the children should expect to do more of the household chores.

23. It's just as important for girls to learn to make repairs around the home as it is for boys.

24. It's just as important for boys to learn to sew as it is for girls.

25. It's important for both boys and girls to learn to use tools.

Suggested Follow-Up:

1. Summarize data:
   a. Male vs. Female
   b. Only child vs. all male vs. all female vs. both male and female
   c. One parent family or two parent family
2. Discuss differences of opinions.
3. Discuss why household chores are seen as male or female jobs.
4. Design computer programs to tap opinions toward occupational roles and recreational activities.

My Family Helps Me — I Help My Family

Concept:

The family serves to perpetuate man and fulfill certain health needs.

General Behavioral Objective:

The student will be able to cite examples of factors contributing to successful family living.

Domain: Affective   *Dimension:* All

Grade Level: Upper elementary

Specific Behavioral Objectives:

1. The student will be able to cite examples of ways the family contributes to personal success by completing the "My Family Helps Me" Worksheet.
2. The student will be able to cite examples of ways he/she contributes to the success of the family by completing the "I Help My Family" Worksheet.

Directions: (Teacher)

1. Duplicate "My Family Helps Me" Worksheet (see p. 170).
2. Duplicate "I Help My Family" Worksheet (see p. 171).

Suggested Follow-Up:

1. Divide class into small groups of 3 or 4 students.
2. Have each group devise and act out a skit demonstrating one of the eight factors listed in the headings of the two worksheets.

"My Family Helps Me" Worksheet

Directions:

1. Each person's family helps to make him/her the successful person he/she is.
2. Think of all the ways your family has helped to bring you to where you are today.
3. Fill out the chart by listing four examples of ways your family has helped you under each of the four headings.

"I Help My Family" Worksheet

Directions:

1. A family is successful when each of its members does his/her best to help.
2. Think of the many ways you are helping your family to be successful.
3. Fill out the chart by listing four examples of ways you are helping your family to be successful under each of the four headings.

MY FAMILY HELPS ME BY . . .

They show they love and care for me by:	They set a good example for me by:
1.	1.
2.	2.
3.	3.
4.	4.

They help me to learn by:	They encourage and support me by:
1.	1.
2.	2.
3.	3.
4.	4.

I HELP MY FAMILY BY . . .

I show love and care for others in the family by:	I set a good example for others by:
1.	1.
2.	2.
3.	3.
4.	4.
I share the workload by:	I try to make them proud of me by:
1.	1.
2.	2.
3.	3.
4.	4.

Yarn Cards

Concept:

The family serves to perpetuate man and fulfill certain health needs.

General Behavioral Objective:

The student will be able to identify the human reproductive organs.

Domain: Cognitive   *Dimension:* Mental

Grade Level: Upper elementary

Specific Behavioral Objective:

The student will be able to identify the male and female pelvic and reproductive organs by using yarn cards.

Directions: (Teacher)

Note: This method is excellent for students on an individual basis, as a self-testing technique. Yarn cards can be developed for any anatomical structure.

1. Choose pieces of heavy, white cardboard approximately 7½″ × 10″. The inside portion of transparency frames is ideal.
2. Draw, one on each card, the following:
   a. Male pelvic and reproductive organs, side view
   b. Female pelvic and reproductive organs, side view
   c. Female reproductive organs, front view.
3. Outline drawings in black felt-tip pen and color organs in various shades.
4. Print the names of the organs to be identified on either side of the drawing. Include in parentheses the phonetic pronounciations for these parts. Avoid placing the name of the organ in close proximity to its part on the drawing.
5. Laminate cards at this point. Since students will use the yarn cards on an individual basis, they will get hard usage. Lamination will help insure protection for future utilization.
6. On outside edge of card, in line with the names of the organs, cut small v-shaped slits, only deep and wide enough for the yarn strings to fit in and be held securely.
7. Make holes large enough for yarn to be pulled through in the organs to be identified. Insert pieces of different colored yarns in each hole. Make sure yarn strings are long enough to reach any of the slits on the card. Then tie the yarn with a knot on the back of the card.
8. Snip additional 1″ pieces of each colored yarn. On the back of the card, attach these in line with the slits in their correct positions with trans-

parent tape. *Be sure that the yarn colors from the drawings correspond with the yarn colors of the correct term.* This will enable the student to tuck the yarn from the drawing into the slit next to the identifying word. If it matches the color of yarn on the back of the card, the student will know that answer is correct.

Directions: (Student)

1. Identify the different parts of the male and female reproductive and pelvic organs by putting the yarn from the organs into the slits by the correct word or term.

2. When you finish, turn the card over. If the color of the pieces of yarn you have put in the slits matches the pieces of yarn on the back of the card, you know you are correct.

3. If you have missed some of the answers, detach all pieces of yarn and try again.

Suggested Follow-Up:

To further reinforce the learning of the parts and functions of the reproductive organs, use the "Scrambled Word" method.

1. Provide a worksheet with the following:
   a. *Column 1* — List the terms with letters scrambled and provide a place for students to rearrange them correctly.
   b. *Column 2* — Have students tell if the organ is part of the male, female, or both reproductive systems.
   c. *Column 3* — Using resource materials, have students describe the function of each organ listed.

Super Series

Concept:

The family serves to perpetuate man and fulfill certain health needs.

General Behavioral Objective:

The student will be able to demonstrate an understanding of the terminology of human reproduction.

Domain: Cognitive   *Dimension:* Mental

Grade Level: Upper elementary

Specific Behavioral Objective:

When given the definition of a term related to human reproduction, the student will be able to indicate verbally the correct word while competing in the "Super Series" game.

Directions: (Teacher)

1. On chalkboard, with masking tape (or chalk), construct or draw a large baseball diamond.

2. Cut out, from different colored pieces of construction paper, two 4″ circles to represent baseballs. Use felt tip pen markings to indicate the stitching on the balls.

3. If the chalkboard is magnetic, place two small pieces of magnetic tape on the back of each baseball. If the chalkboard is not magnetized, use chalk markings to indicate the progress of the game.

4. With chalk, draw a scoreboard similar to those used in a real baseball game, and mark as many innings on it as you wish the game to last.

5. Prepare a series of terms related to human reproduction. On individual 3″ × 5″ cards, print the definitions of the terms on one side. On the opposite side, print the terms defined and their phonetic pronounciation symbols. Laminate the cards.

6. Divide class into two teams — one team sitting on one side of the room, the other team on the other side. Call the teams the "Blue Sox" and the "Yellow Sox" — according to the color of the baseballs used to represent them.

7. Appoint one student to be the umpire and one to be the scorekeeper. Announce their duties to the class:

   a. Umpire:

   1. sees that each student takes turn in order.

   2. holds the pack of cards from which a player not at bat draws the top card.

   3. indicates when an out is charged to a team for talking out of order or aiding a student in answering a question.

   b. Scorekeeper:

   1. marks the progress of the ball from base to base.

   2. keeps track of outs and runs on chalkboard.

   3. fills in scoreboard with the number of runs scored by a team in each half-inning.

Directions: (Student)

1. This game is called "Super Series" and it is played almost like baseball.

2. The object of the game is to score more runs than your opponents.

3. How do you score runs?

   a. Each time one of the players on your team answers correctly, your team baseball, which starts at home plate at the beginning of the inning, advances one base. This is called a hit.

b. Each time the baseball circles the bases and arrives back at home plate (4 hits), your team scores a run. Try to score as many runs as you can before your team makes three outs.

4. How do you make an out?

a. By giving an incorrect answer.

b. By saying, "I do not know."

c. By talking out of order.

d. By helping a teammate with an answer.

5. How do you play the game?

a. When your team is at bat:

1. You will each take turns trying to give the correct word for the definition read to you by the opposing team.

2. Your team stays at bat until three outs are made.

b. When the other team is at bat:

1. You will each take turns reading a definition to your opponents. (The correct answer is on the opposite side of the card.) Draw the top card from the pack held by the umpire.

6. Remember! If you talk out of turn or help your teammate, the umpire will call an out against your team!

7. Play ball!

---

concept 7:

Personal Health Practices are Affected by a Complexity of Forces, Often Conflicting.

Introduction to Concept — Lower Elementary Level

DO YOU SOMETIMES WISH . . .?

Robbie never has to wash his hands before eating. As a matter of fact, he doesn't have to eat all those vegetables or fruits or meats or even drink milk to be strong. He doesn't have to wash behind his ears or scrub his fingernails. He couldn't possibly brush or floss his teeth. Robbie doesn't know how to lie down and sleep, and when he is sick he doesn't have to take medicine to help him to get well.

Do you sometimes wish that you didn't have to do these things? Do you sometimes wish that your mother or father would quit bugging you about these things? Do you wish that you were like Robbie?

Can you guess what Robbie really is?

Here is a picture of Robbie.

Yes, Robbie is a Robot. Now let's go on and see if you still wish you were Robbie.

Here is a "yes or no" test to see what you know about Robbie the Robot. I will read you a sentence and you answer "yes" if you think it is right. If you think the sentence is wrong, answer "no."

1. Robbie Robot is made of pieces of metal and shaped and fitted together.
2. Robbie is alive.
3. Robbie can laugh when he is happy and cry when he is sad or hurt.
4. When someone takes his hand to help him, Robbie feels warm and good.
5. Robbie only moves when someone else makes him do it.
6. Robbie has friends and playmates.
7. Robbie loves hamburgers and French fries.
8. Once in a while Robbie's parts may need oiling, or he may need a new battery.
9. Robbie has to take baths and brush his teeth.
10. He needs clean air to breathe and clothes to keep him warm.
11. Robbie has a mother and father who love him very much.
12. I wish I were Robbie the Robot.
13. I'm glad I am me.

You and I are living, human beings. We can't be turned in for a new model every few years as we do with a car or a refrigerator. Our body is the only one we'll ever have. So we must learn to take care of our bodies, learn everything we can, and learn how to get along with others in order to be as healthy and as happy as possible.

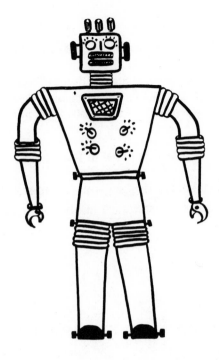

Yes, Robbie is a Robot. Now let's go and see if you still wish you were Robbie.

Paste A Label in The Box

Concept:

Personal health practices are affected by a complexity of forces, often conflicting.

General Behavioral Objective:

The student will be able to cite examples of behaviors that influence personal health.

Domain: Cognitive   *Dimension:* Physical

Grade Level: Lower elementary

Specific Behavioral Objective:

From a list of health behaviors, the student will be able to select ten that help maintain physical health.

Directions: (Teacher)

Prepare a "Staying Healthy Box" worksheet and labels (see pp. 178 and 179).

Suggested Follow-Up:

1. Have students suggest additional good/bad health practices. Write these on the chalkboard.
2. Give each student another "Staying Healthy" worksheet.
3. From the ones written on the chalkboard, have students select behaviors that help people to stay healthy and print them in the empty spaces.

Paste A Label in the Box

Directions:

1. Choose 10 labels of things people do to stay healthy.
2. Cut them out and paste each in one of the boxes below.

THE STAYING HEALTHY BOX

LABELS

Staying up late	Eating fruits and vegetables
Brushing and flossing teeth	Running, jumping, and playing
Eating candy	Watching TV after school and after supper
Washing hands before eating and after bathroom	Washing, brushing, combing hair
Forgetting to brush and floss teeth	Keeping ears warm and clean
Having dirty fingernails	Wearing clean clothes
Getting plenty of sleep	Picking nose
Holding back going to the bathroom	Taking baths
Eating a good breakfast	Chewing a pencil

Vertical Wall Hanging

Concept:

Personal health practices are affected by a complexity of forces, often conflicting.

General Behavioral Objective:

The student will be able to evaluate personal health habits.

Domain: Psychomotor   *Dimension:* Physical

Grade Level: Lower elementary

Specific Behavioral Objective:

After generating a class list of habits conducive to good physical health, the student will be able to construct a vertical wall hanging of four habits needing improvement.

Directions: (Teacher)
1. Cut enough colored construction paper into 4½″ × 5″ pieces for each student to have four different colored pieces.
2. Cut enough 36″ lengths of colored yarn for each student to have one to which he/she can attach finished pieces.
3. Give directions to students verbally.

Directions: (Student — Verbal)

1. A habit is something you do over and over without thinking about it. There are many habits you should practice in order to stay healthy. Can you tell us what some of these habits are? (Teacher: Write these on chalkboard.)
2. Look at the list and pick out *four* health habits in which you need improvement.
3. On each of your colored pieces of paper write one of these health habits you want to improve.
4. Attach your pieces of paper to the yarn by putting a little bit of paste down the middle of the back side.

Suggested Follow-Up:
1. Discuss why the habits selected were chosen.
2. Take wall hanging home and display it where it will serve as a reminder.

My Health — My Feelings

Concept:

Personal health practices are affected by a complexity of forces, often conflicting.

General Behavioral Objective:

The student will be able to evaluate personal feelings about personal health.

Domain: Affective   *Dimension:* Emotional

Grade Level: Lower elementary

Specific Behavioral Objective:

By values voting, the student will be able to indicate the feelings about a series of situations which can affect personal health.

Directions: (Teacher)

1. On pieces of like-sized tagboard make faces demonstrating happiness, anger, love/like, fear, and hurt. Below each face print the appropriate title (see p. 181).
2. Place the faces on the floor in various parts of the room.
3. Direct students to move to the face that best describes their feelings.

FACES OF FEELINGS

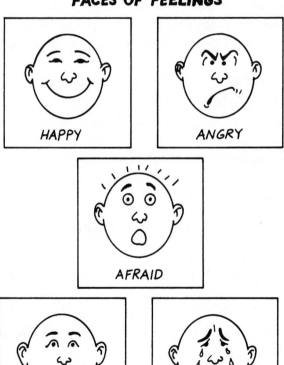

4. Read each situation to students (see p. 182).
5. Stop after each statement is read and have students volunteer to explain why they feel the way they do.
6. Emphasize:
   a. that each person's feeling is OK.
   b. that we have different feelings about the same event.

SITUATIONS

1. When the dentist tells me I have no cavities, I feel . . .
2. When the dentist tells me I should stop eating candy, I feel . . .
3. When my parents take me to the doctor, I feel . . .
4. When my parents make me go to bed but allow my older brother/sister to stay up, I feel . . .
5. When I see someone sneezing without covering his/her mouth and nose, I feel . . .
6. When my parents make me eat my vegetables, I feel . . .
7. When my mother makes me wear my boots to school, I feel . . .
8. When someone tells me I look nice, I feel . . .
9. When my teacher tells me to sit up in my chair, I feel . . .
10. When my parents tell me I can't wear my blue jeans, I feel . . .
11. When someone tells me that I have nice manners, I feel . . .
12. When I am sick and must stay home from school, I feel . . .
13. If someone tells me I'm too fat or too skinny, I feel . . .

I Know Me — I Can Help Me

Concept:

Personal health practices are affected by a complexity of forces, often conflicting.

General Behavioral Objective:

The student will be able to identify behaviors that influence personal health.

Domain: Cognitive   *Dimension:* Physical

Grade Level: Lower elementary

Specific Behavioral Objective:

After drawing specified parts of the body, the student will be able to identify the part affected by a particular health behavior by matching.

Directions: (Teacher)

    1. Prepare worksheets 1 and 2 (see pp. 184 and 185).

Suggested Follow-Up:

    1. Draw a self-portrait doing the one thing you most like to do.

    2. Under the picture, list the parts of the body needed to do the activity.

    3. Discuss what effect it would have if each of the parts were weak or missing.

    4. Verbally complete the sentence:

    In order to be able to do the things I want to do, I must . . .

I KNOW ME — I CAN HELP ME

Directions:

    1. In each of the eight balloons on your worksheet there is a space for you to draw *one* of these things. Can you . . .

      a. Draw your two *ears*?

      b. Draw your *nose*?

      c. Draw your mouth showing your *teeth*?

      d. Draw your two *eyes*? Color them your color.

      e. Draw your finger showing your *fingernail*?

      f. Draw your *hands*?

      g. Draw your *hair*? Color it your color.

      h. Draw your arm showing your *muscle*?

    2. At the end of the string on your balloon, label the picture with the word underlined in the direction.

    3. Now do Worksheet #2.

What Should I WEAR WHERE?

Concept:

    Personal health practices are affected by a complexity of forces, often conflicting.

General Behavioral Objective:

    The student will be able to indicate choices of health practices in a variety of social environments.

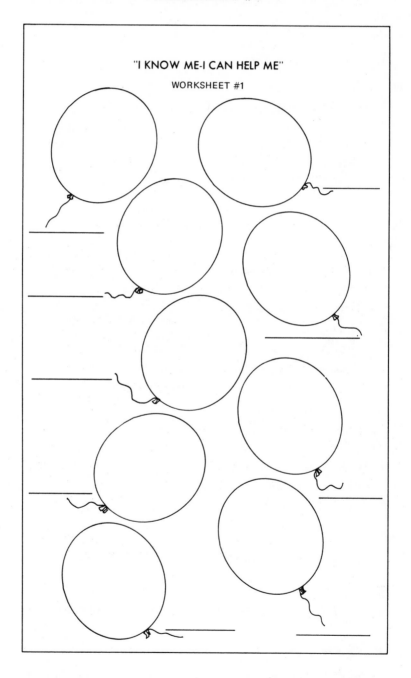

WORKSHEET #2

Directions:

Using the words at the ends of the strings of your balloons, fill in the blanks of these sentences correctly.

1. Sitting too close to the TV is bad for my _____.

2. Exercising helps to make my _____ strong.

3. After going to the bathroom, I should wash my _____.

4. Germs can grow under my _____.

5. I should cover my _____ when I sneeze.

6. Eating too much candy can make my _____ decay.

7. My _____ looks and feels better when I wash, comb, and brush it often.

8. Listening to loud noises for a long time can be bad for my _____.

Domain: Affective   *Dimension:* Social

Grade Level: Lower elementary

Specific Behavioral Objective:

Given a list of social environments, the student will be able to indicate verbally a personal choise of clothing to wear.

Directions: (Student)

What types of clothing would you choose to wear to these social events:

1. A friend's birthday party
2. The local hamburger stand
3. A family picnic
4. Church
5. A football game
6. A friend's home for dinner
7. A nice restaurant (with your family)
8. A school play
9. A movie
10. Playing outdoors with friends in cold weather

Suggested Follow-Up:

1. Student draws a picture of himself/herself, in one of these social situations, wearing the clothing of his/her choice.
2. Discussion of:
   a. Why do we wear clothing?
   b. Why do we choose certain clothing to wear?

Alternative Activity:

1. Cut and mount pictures from magazines depicting the social events.
2. Show the pictures instead of giving them verbally.

---

concept 7:

Personal Health Practices are Affected by a
Complexity of Forces, Often Conflicting.

Introduction to the Concept — Upper Elementary Level

THE WISH

"Wash your hands before eating!"

"Did you brush and floss your teeth?"

"Put on your boots, It's raining hard!"

"Cover your mouth when you sneeze, and use your tissues!"

"But you must take a bath and wash your hair. You've been playing hard all day."

"Turn down the radio. Too much noise is not good for you!"

"Get further back from the TV! It isn't wise to sit too close."

"Pick up your toys and put them where they belong!"

"Eat your vegetables or you won't get dessert!"

"Don't play in the street."

"Time for bed! I don't care if you want to watch the movie! You must get your sleep!"

"Don't put your fingers in your mouth!"

"Don't run when you are carrying scissors!"

"Orders, orders, orders," Jeff thought. "I am so tired of hearing people always telling me what I can and can't do, what I should do, and what I shouldn't do. If I had a wish that could come true, it would be that I didn't have to obey any of the orders people give me!"

Do you ever feel like Jeff is feeling? Can you tell me what might happen in each of these situations if Jeff's wish *did* come true. Let's start with the first one . . .

PRODUCT ELIMINATION GAME

Concept:

Personal health practices are affected by a complexity of forces, often conflicting.

General Behavioral Objective:

The student will be able to evaluate products used in personal health practices.

Domain: Affective   *Dimension:* Physical

Grade Level: Upper elementary

Specific Behavioral Objective:

When given a list of health products, the student will be able to evaluate the importance of each product to his/her personal health practices by rank ordering.

Directions: (Teacher)

1. Prepare and give to students this list of (12) health products commonly used in personal health practices:

   a. soap   g. toothpaste
   b. deodorant   h. towel
   c. shampoo   i . toilet
   d. comb or brush   j . wash cloth
   e. toilet paper   k. bathtub/shower
   f. toothbrush   l . wash machine

2. Have students evaluate each product's importance to him/her. Read these directions to them.

Directions: (Student)

1. Read through your list.

2. Decide which product you could most easily do without. Place a #1 in front of the product in your list.

3. Decide which product you could next most easily do without, and place a #2 beside it.

To Teacher: Continue this process through #12.

4. Will you share with us what you had and why for #1? #2? #3? #10? #11? #12?

Suggested Follow-Up:

1. On the chalkboard make a graph of products which could most/least be done without.

Product	1	2	3	10	11	12
Soap						
Deodorant						
Shampoo						
Comb/Brush						
Toilet Paper						
Toothbrush						
Toothpaste						
Towel						
Toilet						
Medicine						
Bathtub/Shower						
Wash Machine						

2. Discuss reasons for selection.

A Tisket, A Tasket!
What's In The Dental Health Basket?

(ACTIVITY 1)

Concept:

Personal health practices are affected by a complexity of forces, often conflicting.

General Behavioral Objective:

The student will be able to identify words related to dental health.

Domain: Cognitive   *Dimension:* Physical

Grade Level: Upper elementary

Specific Behavioral Objective:

Given a worksheet containing a variety of words, the student will be able to identify the 17 related to dental health by writing the definitions.

Directions: (Teacher)

1. Duplicate Worksheets 1 and 2 for each student (see pp. 190 and 191).
2. Provide resource materials from the American Dental Association.
3. Dental Health words in list:

Toothbrush	Plaque
Toothpaste	Floss
Drill	Carbohydrates
Dentist	Gingivitis
Orthodontist	Bacteria
Caries	Acid
Pyorrhea	Filling
Fluoride	Disclosing tablets
Gums	

Introduction:

Very few people go through life without tooth decay. Without proper care of your teeth now and throughout your life, you may be one of the people who will suffer from serious gum disease. Some of you will even lose all of your teeth.

189

A Tisket, A Tasket! What's in the Dental Health Basket?

DIRECTIONS:

1. The "Dental Health Basket" contains many different words. Some of these are words you need to know when you learn about dental health.

2. Find the 17 words important to dental health.

3. Write those you find on worksheet 2. Then write the definition for each.

4. Use the materials on the resource table.

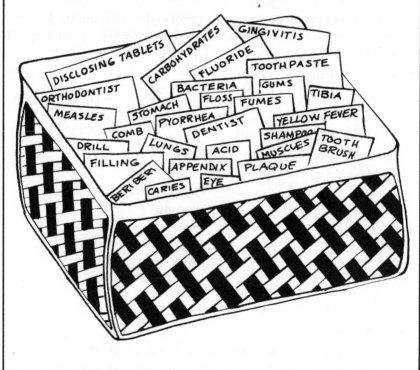

In order to understand about dental health, there are some words you must know and understand.

Suggested Follow-Up:

    1. "A Tisket, A Tasket! What's in The Dental Health Basket?" Activity 2.

    2. Include vocabulary words in spelling lesson.

Worksheet 2

Word	Definition
1.	1.
2.	2.
3.	3.
4.	4.
5.	5.
6.	6.
7.	7.
8.	8.
9.	9.
10.	10
11.	11.
12.	12.
13.	13.
14.	14.
15.	15.
16.	16.
17.	17.

A Tisket, A Tasket! What's In the Dental Health Basket?

ACTIVITY 2

Concept:

Personal health practices are affected by a complexity of forces, often conflicting.

General Behavioral Objective:

The student will be able to identify words related to dental health.

Domain: Cognitive   *Dimension:* Physical

Grade Level: Upper elementary

Specific Behavioral Objective:

Given clues, the student will be able to identify seventeen terms related to dental health by unscrambling the letters.

Directions: (Teacher)

1. Duplicate Activity 2 worksheet (see p. 192-194).

Suggested Follow-Up:

1. Utilize curricular materials from the American Dental Association.
2. Supplementary curricular materials to implement the ADA program for K-2-5 are also available from Metropolitan Health Planning Corporation, 908 Standard Building, Cleveland, Ohio 44113.

ACTIVITY 2 WORKSHEET

Directions:

1. Unscramble the letters to correctly spell the word(s). These are the same words you had in the learning activity before.
2. Use the clues given. They will help!

1. t o t o r n s d t h i o

   _ _ _ _ _ _ _ _ _ _ _

   A dentist who fits bands on teeth to move them into their correct position.

2. o b t u r h s t o h

   _ _ _ _ _ _ _ _ _

   You put toothpaste on this.

3. i d l l r

   _ _ _ _ _

   What the dentist uses to remove decay before filling a tooth.

4. l n f g i i l

   _ _ _ _ _ _ _

   What the dentist puts into a decayed tooth after cleaning it out.

5. t e i d t s n

— — — — — — —

A person who examines and cares for teeth.

6. i a e c r s

— — — — — —

Another name for tooth decay.

7. r p e r a h o y

— — — — — — — —

An infection of the gums caused by not caring for the teeth.

8. f o l i r u e d

— — — — — — — —

A chemical (KEH-mihkul) that helps prevent tooth decay.

9. u m s g

— — — —

The part of the mouth around the bottom of the teeth.

10. l q p u e a

— — — — — —

A sticky, almost invisible film that clings to the surface of a tooth.

11. l s o s f

— — — — —

String-like material that can help remove trapped food particles and plaque from between-the teeth.

12. b h r c e y o s t a a r d

— — — — — — — — — — —

The family of foods to which sugar belongs. They are your teeth's worst enemies.

13. l d g i s c n s i o   (two words)
    b e a t t l

— — — — — — — — — —

— — — — — —

A colored wafer you put in your mouth and chew that shows you where there is plaque on your teeth.

14. i v g i n i s t g i

— — — — — — — — —

When gums become reddened and painful because of improper care.

15. t b a e a i r c

— — — — — — — —

Tiny germs in plaque that combine with carbohydrates to form an acid that causes teeth to decay.

16. o t b h o h s t r u

— — — — — — — — —

What you use every day to remove food particles from your teeth and to polish them.

17. d c i a

— — — —

What forms on your teeth when carbohydrates combine with bacteria.

What's The Problem?

Concept:

Personal health practices are affected by a complexity of forces, often conflicting.

General Behavioral Objective:

The student will be able to discuss the consequences of poor health practices.

Domain: Affective   *Dimension:* All

Grade Level: Upper elementary

Specific Behavioral Objective:

Given a series of behaviors, the students, in small groups, will be able verbally to suggest possible causes and consequences.

Directions: (Teacher)

1. It is assumed that students understand that all behaviors have causes, consequences, and alternatives.

2. Organize students into small groups of four or five. Have them choose a recorder to write down the group's suggestions.

3. Prepare a worksheet for each small group (see p. 195).

Suggested Follow-Up:

1. Recorders report the group findings to the class.

2. Discuss the possible causes and consequences.

"WHAT'S THE PROBLEM?" WORKSHEET

Directions:

1. Discuss each of these situations carefully.

2. Suggest as many answers to each question as possible.

3. Recorder: Write down answers the group comes up with.

Situations:

1. *Terry comes to school dirty almost every morning.*
   a. What do you think might be causing this?
   b. What might happen to Terry because of this?
   c. What might Terry do to solve this problem?

2. *Jackie falls asleep in class almost every day.*
   a. Why might this be happening?
   b. What might happen to Jackie because of this?
   c. What might Jackie do to solve the problem?

3. *Kim uses lunch money to buy desserts, french fries, and after-school candy.*
   a. Why do you think Kim is doing this?
   b. What might happen to Kim because of this?
   c. What should Kim do instead of this?

4. *Jamie refuses to go to the dentist.*
   a. What might be the cause of this?
   b. What may happen to Jamie because of this?
   c. What could Jamie do about this?

5. *Toni's grades are going down.*
   a. Why might this be happening?
   b. What might happen to Toni because of this?
   c. What might Toni do to solve the problem?

6. *Dana's stomach growls from hunger about an hour after getting to school.*
   a. What might be the cause of this?
   b. What might happen to Dana because of being hungry?
   c. What might Dana do to solve the problem?

concept 8:

Utilization of Health Information, Products, and Services is Guided by Values and Perceptions

Introduction to Concept — Lower Elementary Level

AUNT TILL'S PILLS

It seemed that Aunt Till had a cure for almost anything. She had appointed herself as chief doctor for the family. It didn't matter if someone was overweight, underweight, had a stomachache, earache, toothache, legache, backache — any kind of ache or pain. Aunt Till knew what the trouble was, and *she* had the cure.

She had brightly colored pills in all sizes and shapes, bottles of stuff you could swallow from a spoon, creamy lotions, and stinging ointments to rub on any part of the body when it hurt or needed care. She even had all sorts of electric gadgets she would use to try to help someone feel better.

Aunt Till's bathroom looked like a small drug store. When the medicine chest could no longer hold the things, she had new shelves built. Anytime a new medicine, skin cream, deodorant — any kind of health product — was advertised on television or in newspapers and magazines, Aunt Till felt she *had* to buy it. She told everyone that it was silly to go to a doctor, since she knew what was wrong and what would cure it. That was, until Aunt Till herself became very sick.

She took the red pills, the white pills, the green capsules — every color and shape of pill she had. She swallowed the syrupy medicines and rubbed her aching body with the different ointments. She used a heating pad, an ice pack, and all the machines she had tucked away in the closet. But Aunt Till's illness got worse and worse.

It wasn't until she became so sick that she couldn't get out of bed that Aunt Till allowed the family to call Doctor Smith. The doctor discovered what was wrong with Aunt Till and started her on the road to recovery. It took many months for her to get back to being her old self. Well, almost her old self!

196

There was one big change in Aunt Till. Her medicine chest and shelves are now almost empty. The pills and medicines and ointments are no longer there. The electrical gadgets are gathering dust in the attic. She no longer tries to treat others for their illnesses. Instead, she tells them to visit their doctor. Aunt Till had learned a big lesson. Can you guess what that lesson was?

The answer is simple. Dr. Smith told her that if she had called sooner, the cure could have started earlier and she would not have suffered so much. Now Aunt Till realizes that, even though doctors can't cure every illness, they know more about illnesses and cures than she does.

Do you know someone like Aunt Till?

Can you draw a picture of Aunt Till's medicine chest and shelves before she learned her lesson?

Health Products are for People

Concept:

Utilization of health information, products, and services is guided by values and perceptions.

General Behavioral Objective:

The student will be able to discriminate between health and nonhealth products.

Domain: Cognitive   *Dimension:* Mental

Grade Level: Lower elementary

Specific Behavioral Objective:

When given a series of descriptions of behaviors involving health and nonhealth products, the student will be able to identify the health products by circling the correct words.

Directions: (Teacher)

 1. Prelearning: definition for the term *health product.*
    a. What is a health product?
    b. Put the correct definition on a piece of tagboard. Affix pieces of magnetic tape to the back and display the definition on the chalkboard. (If the chalkboard is not magnetized use masking tape.)
    c. Read the definition in unison.
    DEFINITION: A health product (PRAH-dukt) is something made by a company, other than food, that people use to protect (proh-TEKT) and promote (proh-MOHT) (make better) their health.
 2. Duplicate and distribute the "Health Products are for People" Worksheet (see p. 199).
 3. Read directions to students.

4. Key:
1. toothbrush, toothpaste
2. glasses
3. none
4. washcloth, soap, towel
5. none
6. leg braces
7. none
8. bandage
9. medicine
10. shampoo
11. hearing aid
12. none
13. bands
14. brush, comb

Suggested Follow-Up:

1. Identify things in the sentences that are nonhealth products and explain why.
2. Draw a picture of each of the health products he/she uses before coming to school.

Where Did You Find Out That . . .?

Concept:

Utilization of health information, products, and services is guided by values and perceptions.

General Behavioral Objective:

The student will be able to identify sources of health information.

Domain: Cognitive   *Dimension:* Mental

Grade Level: Lower elementary

Specific Behavioral Objective:

On a health information checklist, the student will be able to identify personal sources of the health information.

Directions: (Teacher)

Prepare checklist as per p. 200.

Introduction/Discussion:

Every year you learn more and more about ways you can protect or improve your health. We call all of these things "health information". You use this health information every day of your life.

Can you tell us what health information you have used today to help you to stay well?

"HEALTH PRODUCTS ARE FOR PEOPLE" WORKSHEET

Directions:

1. Find the health products in some of the sentences below.
2. When you find a health product, put a circle around it.
3. Not all sentences have health products in them. Some sentences have more than one. BE CAREFUL.
4. If you are not yet sure what a health product is, study the definition again.

Statements:

1. I use a toothbrush and toothpaste to brush my teeth.

2. Some people wear glasses to help them to see better.

3. I like to drink fruit juice for breakfast.

4. When bathing or showering, I use a washcloth, soap, and towel.

5. I like to sit in a comfortable chair to watch television.

6. Johnny must wear leg braces so that he can walk.

7. Hamburgers are my favorite food.

8. My mother put a bandage on my cut finger.

9. When I am sick, the doctor gives me medicine to help me feel better.

10. I like to feel the suds from the shampoo when I wash my hair.

11. My grandmother wears a hearing aid to help her to hear better.

12. I ride to school on a school bus.

13. Susie wears bands on her teeth to help them to grow straight.

14. My hair looks better if I use a brush or comb.

You have learned your health information in many different ways. Can you tell us where you learned some of the ways you know to keep healthy?

Even though people have health information, they sometimes do not use it.

Can you think of some things you know you ought to do to stay healthy, but don't?

Today you are going to check out where you first learned some of your health information.

Suggested Follow-Up:

    1. Identify the "other sources" and develop a listing of "Sources of Health Information".

"WHERE DID YOU FIND OUT THAT . . .?" CHECKLIST

Directions:

    1. Read each statement in the checklist.

    2. Put a check (✓) in the box that tells where you *first* learned the information in the statement.

Health Information	Learned from:				
	Family	Friends	School	T.V.	Other Place
1. Some chewing gum has no sugar in it					
2. Tooth paste with fluoride in it helps to prevent tooth decay					
3. Some shampoos do not hurt when the suds get into the eyes					
4. Everything said about health products in T.V. commercials isn't true					
5. The purpose of commercials is to sell something					

Health Protectors

Concept:

Utilization of health information, products, and services is guided by values and perceptions.

General Behavioral Objective:

The student will be able to identify people who promote and protect physical health.

Domain: Cognitive   *Dimension:* Physical

Grade Level: Lower elementary

Specific Behavioral Objective:

Given a series of pictures and descriptions of people who promote and protect health, the student will be able to identify each by circling the correct answer.

Directions: (Teacher)

1. Duplicate and distribute the "Health Protectors" Worksheet (see p. 202).
2. Read directions to the students.

Directions: (Students)

1. Look carefully at each of the pictures.

2. Think about what the person in the picture is trying to do.

3. Read the description of the person's job below the picture.

4. Circle the correct answer from those given.

Suggested Follow-Up:

1. Discussion:
   a. What else do these Health Protectors do to help us?
   b. Who else in our community are Health Protectors?

HEALTH PROTECTORS WORKSHEET

1.

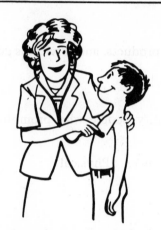

I HELP PEOPLE WHO ARE ILL
I AM A...
FIREMAN
POLICE OFFICER
DOCTOR
DENTIST

2.

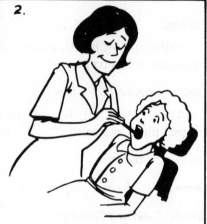

I KEEP YOUR TEETH AND
GUMS HEALTHY. I AM A...
NURSE
DENTIST
EYE DOCTOR
FIREMAN

3.

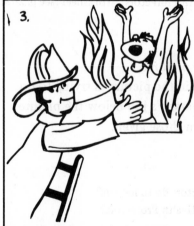

I HELP RESCUE PEOPLE
I AM A...
DENTIST
BABY DOCTOR
NURSE
FIREMAN

4.

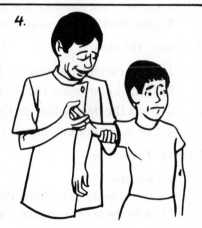

I HELP DOCTORS HELP PEOPLE
I AM A...
NURSE
DOCTOR
DENTIST
POLICE OFFICER

concept 8:

Utilization of Health Information, Products, and
Services Is Guided by Values and Perceptions.

Introduction to Concept — Upper Elementary Level

QUENTIN QUACK

From his name, you might imagine that Quentin Quack is a duck.
But such is not the case. Quentin Quack is the "Chief Product
Pusher" in the Quack family. The Quack family's business is to try
to sell health products to people whether they need them or not.
Sometimes the means they use to do this are not truthful. Sometimes the products they try to sell are not even *good* for people.
The Quack family doesn't worry about this, however, because their
only purpose is to sell products and make lots of money. They have
been in business for a long time, and they are doing very well.

Long ago Quentin discovered that the best way to sell the Quack
family health products was to appeal to people's greatest needs—
to prevent illness, to feel better when ill or bothered, to be attractive and accepted by other people, and, to be successful. He determined that by making health products that promised to fulfill
needs of people (whether they really did or not) and advertising
them wherever and whenever possible, people would spend money to
buy the products. You see, even though he is a cheat, Quentin is a
pretty smart "product pusher."

Day in and day out Quentin is busy inventing medicines, foods, and
machines that *he* says will cure illnesses for which even the greatest
scientists have not discovered causes or cures. He promises all good
things to all people, even though he secretly knows that some of his
products may be dangerous to some people. His only concern is for
the money that will come in so that he can go on inventing new
products and pushing them on the public through his advertisements.

You may have seen some of his advertisements on television, in the
newspapers, magazines, or comic books. His ads are different from
the ordinary ones you might see or hear. You'll know if it is a Quack
family health product if the advertisement for it:

(1) promises a quick cure for a physical or mental ailment, or

(2) describes a case history of someone who has been cured by a product, or

(3) has letters from people telling how successful the product was for them and signed with only the initials of those people, or

(4) claims to have a "secret" ingredient, formula, ray, or

(5) says that doctors won't prescribe the product because they don't want to lose patients, or that they are jealous that someone else discovered the product.

Have you ever really studied advertisements for health products closely?

Have you ever seen or heard an advertisement that might be a "quack product"?

Even though the government has laws and agencies that try to put Quentin Quack and his family out of business, they are not always successful. Until you, and all other people, can spot a "quack" health product, Quentin will go on and on robbing people of both their money and their health.

In what ways do you think quacks can rob you of your health?

Why do you think quacks make so much money?

Can you draw a picture of what you think Quentin Quack looks like doing his thing?

Q.Q. or OK?

Concept:

Utilization of health information, products, and services is guided by values and perceptions.

General Behavioral Objective:

The student will be able to detect examples of possible quack product advertisements.

Domain: Affective   *Dimension:* Mental

Grade Level: Upper elementary

Specific Behavioral Objective:

When given examples of legitimate and possible quack health product advertisements, the student will be able to differentiate between them by categorizing each.

Directions: (Teacher)

1. Cut out samples of both legitimate and quack health product advertisements (see introduction) from magazines and newspapers.
2. Paste each randomly on sheets of colored construction paper and number in sequence.
3. Laminate each sheet of construction paper containing numbered advertisements. This will protect them from destruction and they will be available for future use.
4. Options for learning:
   a. Use as an experience at one of a series of learning stations.
   b. Pass advertisements around for students to identify the advertisements individually.
   c. Have students work in small groups to discuss and categorize each advertisement. When finished with one sheet, they may exchange with another group until all are completed.
   d. Display advertisements on a bulletin board or table for students to examine individually.

Directions: (Student)

1. Number your paper from 1 to ———.
2. Each of these sheets contains a number of advertisements for health products. Some of these are OK and some might be labeled as quack advertisements. In our introduction you learned some of the ways that quacks advertise their health products. If you think that an advertisement is all right, place an "OK" beside the number of the ad on your paper. If you think it is a quack advertisement, place a "QQ" (Quentin Quack) beside the number on your paper.
3. Work until you have examined and completed each advertisement.

Suggested Follow-Up:

1. Have students justify their answers in total classroom discussion. Use criteria from "Quentin Quack".
2. Have pupils cut out and bring in further examples of quack advertising of health products.

Buy My Product Because . . .

Concept:

Utilization of health information, products, and services is guided by values and perceptions.

General Behavioral Objective:

The student will be able to analyze health product advertisements.

Domain: Cognitive   *Dimension:* All

Grade Level: Upper elementary

Specific Behavioral Objective:

When shown a series of health product advertisements, the students, in small groups, will be able to list the emotional, social, or physical appeal used by the advertiser to sell the product.

Directions: (Teacher)

1. Cut out from magazines and newspapers a variety of advertisements for commonly used health products (soaps, deodorants, toothpastes, first-aid products, creams, lotions, laxatives, make-up, shampoos, sleep inducers, antacids, etc.).

2. Make sure that a variety of appeals are represented in the advertisements such as appeals to beauty, glamour, ease of use, cleaner, whiter, relief of pain, relaxation, shinier, masculinity–femininity, money-back guarantees, coupons, free samples, famous person endorsements, graphs, scientific study statistics, extra added ingredient, etc.

3. Mount these on colored construction paper and number each sequentially. Laminate to preserve the advertisements for future use.

4. Organize students in small groups. Give each group several advertisements.

5. Have students list in writing the promises or appeals that the advertiser uses in order to sell his product.

Directions: (Student)

Introduction:

Sometimes there are many health products that can be used for the same purpose such as toothpastes to clean teeth, shampoos to clean hair, soaps to keep the body clean, etc.

A manufacturer of one of these health products must compete with his rivals (other manufacturers of the same kind of product) to try to get people to buy his product rather than one of the others. He does this by advertising the product in magazines, newspapers, on radio, and on television. In his advertisements for his product, the manufacturer tries to make people feel they need to use his product by making promises (appeals) that his product will do certain things better than the products of his rivals. He tries to fulfill people's needs to be attractive to others, to feel better physically and mentally, and to be successful.

1. Appoint a recorder to do the writing for your group.

2. Each of your groups has several advertisements. Study each one carefully. See if you can discover what promises, appeals,

or gimmicks the advertiser is using to try to get the public to buy the product.

3. The recorder will list your findings for each advertisement.

Suggested Follow-Up:

Have recorder for each group display each of his group's advertisements singly and report the findings of the group to the entire class.

Alternative:

1. Use as an activity for Station Learning.

Health Agency Symbols

Concept:

Utilization of health information, products, and services is guided by values and perceptions.

General Behavioral Objective:

The student will be able to identify a variety of community health agencies.

Domain: Cognitive   *Dimension:* Mental

Grade Level: Upper elementary

Specific Behavioral Objective:

When shown the symbols for a variety of community health agencies, the student will be able to identify each by matching.

Directions: (Teacher)

1. Draw the symbols for a number of health service agencies on a ditto master. Omit any lettering that might give a clue to its identity. Suggestions for symbols: American Red Cross, American Cancer Society, American Heart Association, American Lung Association, United Way, American Dental Association, National Safety Council, American Medical Association.
2. Provide the titles for each agency and have students identify the symbol and the agency by matching.

Directions: (Student)

1. There are many places and people you can turn to in order to get good, reliable health information when you need it. Your doctor, your pharmacist, or your local health clinics may be some sources of good information. Others may be certain

health agencies (groups) that research and provide sound
health information to people.

2. On your paper are some common symbols (emblems) of
some health agencies that may be familiar to you. See if you
can match the symbol with the name of the health agency.

Suggested Follow-Up:

1. Choose one of the agencies from the list and write a report describing
the work of that group.

Alternative:

This learning experience may be done in one of a series of learning stations in this concept.

Why Buy?

Concept:

Utilization of health information, products, and services is
guided by values and perceptions.

General Behavioral Objective:

The student will be able to evaluate the personal appeal of health
product promotions.

Domain: Affective   *Dimension:* Emotional, Social

Grade Level: Upper elementary

Specific Behavioral Objective:

Given a series of behavioral statements involving emotional and
social influences, the student will be able to justify the personal
selection or rejection of each influence.

Directions: (Teacher)

Duplicate and distribute the "Why Buy" worksheet (see p. 209–
210).

Suggested Follow-Up:

1. Give the students a list of influences that might persuade them to use
certain health products. Examples: friends, family, TV advertisements,
magazine advertisements, attractive containers, endorsements, etc.
2. Rank order these influences from 1 to _____, with #1 being the in-

fluence that would most persuade them to buy certain products, and # ____ being the least influential in getting them to buy products.

3. Announce results to class.

"WHY BUY?" WORKSHEET

Directions:

1. Read each statement carefully.
2. Circle the answer that best describes your action.
3. Tell why you circled that answer.

1. When I see a product advertised on my favorite television show, I try to get my parent to buy it.

   Yes   Sometimes   No

   Why? _____

2. If a famous person, such as my favorite athlete or movie star, said a product was good, I would want to use it.

   Yes   Sometimes   No

   Why? _____

3. I would choose to buy health products my friends use.

   Yes   Sometimes   No

   Why? _____

4. I would choose to buy health products that come in attractive containers.

   Yes   Sometimes   No

   Why? _____

5. I would choose to use health products other members of my family do.

   Yes   Sometimes   No

   Why? _____

6. If I were to have a choice of health products to buy, I would choose those I am familiar with from advertisements.

   Yes   Maybe   No

   Why?_____

7. I believe that all advertisements are truthful.

   Yes   No

   Why? _____

---

concept 9:

The Use of Substances That Modify Mood and Behavior Arises from a Variety of Motivations.

Introduction to Concept — Lower Elementary Level

Note: The abuse of drugs at the lower elementary level tends to be insignificant. Therefore, the focus at this level for this concept is on providing children with opportunities to share their ideas for dealing with the myriad of new situations inherent to school life. Children need practice in learning to cope with situations that cause them to be concerned or afraid. They need to learn which adults can be trusted and helpful to them when they have problems. They need to develop a sense of their own personal worth.

THE STRANGER

Do you often watch a story on television? Do you sometimes go to the movies with your family or friends? Have you ever seen a play on the stage with real people playing the parts? How many of *you* have ever played a part in a skit or a play? What are the people called who take part in these stories on TV, these movies you watch, or these plays you see?

Would you like to hear a story about an actor? This is the story called *The Stranger.*

You are probably wondering why Sneaky Snatcher is one of the greatest actors ever. Perhaps it is because he can be anywhere in the world at any time. He can be right outside of your school or outside of your home. He may hang around the movie theater, the playground, the shopping center, on brightly lit streets or on lonely roads.

He can be a man or a woman, a boy or a girl. He can be dressed in clothing that is different from any you have seen before, or he can be dressed just like the people you see every day.

Sneaky Snatcher can be tall and skinny, short and fat, or in between. He may have white, red, black, or yellow skin. His face can be ugly or beautiful or neither.

He may pretend to be friendly and warm but he really is not. He even may offer to help you or to give you something that you would really like to have. But he is not doing it because he likes you or thinks you are cool. It is because he is selfish and wants only to do *his* thing. Sneaky Snatcher needs people — especially young people, just like you. The only way you can keep from being hurt by this stranger is to be very, very careful. Is it any wonder that this actor who wears so many masks and acts in so many different ways might be dangerous to you?

Let's learn a song about Sneaky Snatcher.

Sneaky Snatcher

Don Masaitis
Barbara Morrow

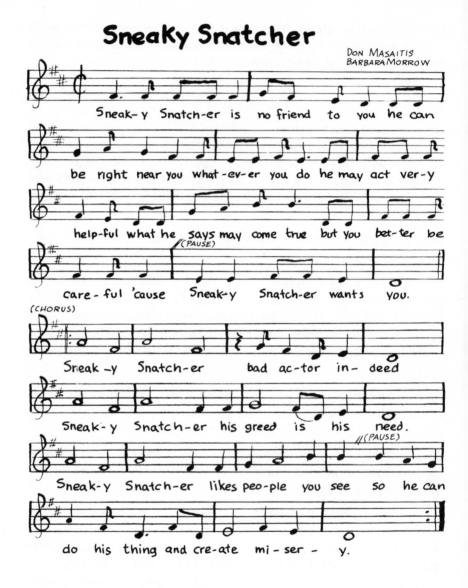

SNEAKY SNATCHER SONG

Sneaky Snatcher is no friend to you.
He can be right near you
Whatever you do.
He may act very helpful,

What he says may sound true.
But you better be careful because
Sneaky Snatcher wants you!

CHORUS
Sneaky Snatcher — bad actor indeed.
Sneaky Snatcher — his greed is his need.
Sneaky Snatcher likes people, you see,
So he can do this thing and create misery.

Can you draw a picture of how you think Sneaky Snatcher looks?

Yes, Yes! No, No!

Concept:

The use of substances that modify mood and behavior arises from a variety of motivations.

General Behavioral Objective:

The student will be able to evaluate behaviors which may either be helpful or harmful to him or to others.

Domain: Affective   *Dimension:* Physical

Grade Level: Lower elementary

Specific Behavioral Objective:

In a large group, the student will be able to determine which of a series of situations would be a threat to personal physical safety by responding verbally with a "yes,yes" or a "no,no."

Introduction:

From our story about *The Stranger*, we know that Sneaky Snatcher can be almost anywhere, anytime. I am going to read some situations to you. If the situation might hurt you, it's a "no,no." If it is a safe situation, it's a "yes, yes." Softly, call out your answer together.

Alternative:

The room may be divided into "yes,yes" and "no,no" sections with the students moving to the side of their choice for each situation.

Situations:

1. Your mother's best friend stops and asks you if you want a ride home from school.
2. You and your older brother are alone in the house. A man comes to the door asking to use the telephone.
3. An older boy hanging around the playground says he has something to show you and wants you to go with him.
4. A kindly-looking old lady offers you a piece of candy.
5. Someone calls on the telephone and asks what your phone number is. You ask what number is being called instead of telling your phone number.
6. A man you have seen, but don't know, offers to take you and your friend to your favorite hamburger place for a sandwich.
7. At night you choose to walk on a well-lighted street instead of taking a short-cut through the woods.
8. You immediately tell your mother when you see your baby brother creeping toward the cupboard that has her household cleaner in it.
9. You love animals. A dog you have never seen before is in your backyard. You run toward him to pet him.
10. You find your favorite candy bar in your Halloween trick-or-treat bag. The wrapper on the candy is loose and partly torn. You decide to throw it away instead of eating it.

Suggested Follow-Up:

1. Discuss why some of the situations could be a threat to their physical safety.
2. Role play Situations 1,2,3,4,6 and 9.

Who Can I Turn To?

Concept:

The use of substances that modify mood and behavior arises from a variety of motivations.

General Behavioral Objective:

The student will be able to decide which people can be most helpful in situations that involve medicines.

Domain: Affective   *Dimension:* Social

Grade Level: Lower elementary

Specific Behavioral Objectives:

1. When given three situations involving the use of medicines, the student will be able to name the people who could be helpful in each situation.
2. Using the list of people identified as helpful, the student will be able to decide how helpful each person could be by rank ordering from most helpful to least helpful.

Directions: (Teacher)

1. Prepare blank ·flash cards with backing to use on an adhesion-board (magnetic chalkboard, felt or flannel board).
2. As answers are given, print flash cards.
3. Arrange flash cards in rank order.
4. Repeat procedure for each situation.

Directions: (Student)

1. After I read a situation to you, tell me who would be able to help you.
2. Now, let's study our list and see how we would rank these people. Which one would be the most helpful to you in this situation? If it weren't possible to ask him/her, who would be your next choice (continue through list)?

Situation 1

Your parents have gone grocery shopping. You and a friend are playing in the house. You find your friend on the bathroom floor with a bottle of your dad's medicine beside him/her. You can't awaken your friend.

Situation 2

You and a friend are walking to the neighborhood park to play. You see a man lying under the bushes who is in pain. When you get closer, he points to his pocket. In his pocket you find a bottle of pills.

Situation 3

It's lunch time at school. John is bragging about how good-tasting his medicine is. Jerry grabs the bottle and drinks the rest of it. During the afternoon recess, Jerry tells you he feels sick and goes to the rest room.

Suggested Follow-Up:

1. Discuss why they chose the people they did after each situation.
2. Discuss why they consider some people to be more helpful than others.

Warning!!

Concept:

The use of substances that modify mood and behavior arises from a variety of motivations.

General Behavioral Objective:

The student will be able to indicate products useful in the home that may be dangerous under certain circumstances.

Domain: Psychomotor   *Dimension:* Physical

Grade Level: Lower elementary

Specific Behavioral Objective:

The student, with parental assistance, will survey and list products commonly used in his/her own home whose labels contain the word "WARNING."

Directions: (Teacher)

1. Students will need to learn the word "WARNING."
2. New vocabulary in the health concepts may be included in spelling lessons.
3. Bring in sample products with labels containing the word "WARNING."

Directions: (Students)

1. When you go home from school today, ask one of your parents to help you look at some of the labels on products used around the house.
2. Make a list of the names of all products that you find that have the word "WARNING" on the label.
3. Bring the list to school tomorrow.

Suggested Follow-Up:

1. Compile a list of all of the products.
2. Discuss proper storage and use of potentially dangerous household products.

3. Develop a display table of empty containers or labels from household products.

---

concept 9:

The Use of Substances that Modify Mood and Behavior Arises from a Variety of Motivations.

Introduction To Concept — Upper Elementary Level

FOLLOW THE LEADER?

I'm thinking of a game that I am sure you have all played or still play once in awhile. In this game one person performs many different actions. You must do these actions exactly as that person does them, or you are out of the game.

Can you guess the name of the game?

Do you remember how the leader did things that were very difficult and sometimes were even dangerous? It didn't matter to you at the time whether the actions were easy to do, hard to do , or dangerous. Your only thought was to prove to others you could do them so that you could stay in the game. Sometimes you were successful. Sometimes you weren't. Sometimes you may have been injured. Sometimes *you* were the leader too.

Did you ever stop to think that you, and everyone else, play the game of "Follow The Leader" every day of your life? Perhaps you don't think of it as being a game, and it really isn't. It's just a part of everyday living. Sometimes you are a follower and sometimes you are a leader in the things you say and do, day in and day out.

Can you think of some ways that you played the role of a *leader* already today?

Can you think of some ways that you played the role of a *follower* today?

Leaders come in two different styles — those who want you to do things because they feel it is best for you and others, and those that want you to do things the way they do even though it may be harmful to you and others. You will always have big decisions to make about which leaders you should follow, whether it be the friends you choose today or the candidate for President you will someday support.

Here are some situations describing some leaders. If you think that they are leaders you *would* choose to imitate or follow, raise your hand and make a fist with your thumb pointing up. If you think the action of the leaders in the situations might be harmful to you and others and you *would not* choose to follow or support them, raise your hand and make a fist with your thumb pointing down. If you are not sure of your answer, fold your arms over your chest.

Note to Teacher:

Discuss answers after each situation.

SITUATIONS

1. Kenny Kool thinks he is a big shot because he smokes cigarettes. He tries to talk you into doing it. You would like to look cool too.
2. Mother insists that you take the medicine that the doctor gave you for your illness. You hate the taste of it!
3. There are some kids in your neighborhood who have a club that you would like to join. You know, however, that in order to join you must be able to shoplift successfully an article from the local discount store.
4. The teacher invites you to stay after school to get some extra help in a subject in which you are doing poorly.
5. In school there is a small group that beats up on other kids to get their lunch money. They want you to join.
6. Juan is a new student in your class. The teacher wants you to help him with his assignments because he has difficulty understanding the language.
7. Your physical education teacher tells you that you are very skilled in a certain activity. He/she wants you to practice everyday at home and follow some training rules.

8. There has been a great deal of crime in your town. The mayor wants all people under 16 years of age to be off the streets by 9:00 PM unless they are with adults.

9. Ann's grandmother says that everyone should take a laxative once a week.

10. Your big brother makes model airplanes and uses smelly glue to put them together. Your friend stays with you one night and wants you both to try sniffing the glue.

One of the most important life decisions you are going to have to make concerns the use of drugs, alcohol, and tobacco. That's what you are going to be learning about in this concept. Follow the leader? It's up to you.

Habits: Easy to Make — Hard to Break

Concept:

The use of substances that modify mood and behavior arises from a variety of motivations.

General Behavioral Objective:

The student is able to analyze reasons why smoking becomes habitual and a threat to future health.

Domain: Cognitive   *Dimension:* Mental

Grade Level: Upper elementary

Specific Behavioral Objective 1:

After completing a stem sentence, the student will be able to define the term "habit" through class consensus.

Introduction:

Most of us have someone in our lives whom we admire and like so much that we think we would like to be just like him/her. Some of these people are in our own family, some are not. Some are our friends, others may be famous people. We try to copy the way that person dresses, talks, acts, walks, eats, and even some of the habits that person has. Think about the person you admire and want to be like the most. Have you ever tried to copy that person in any way?

Will you share with the class the ways you have tried to copy this person? You need not tell us who that person is.

Directions: (Student)

1. In your own words complete this sentence in writing: A habit is . . .
2. Share your answer with the total class.
3. As a class, vote on the definition which would be most acceptable to you.

Domain: Affective   *Dimension:* All

Specific Behavioral Objective 2:

On the chart provided, the student will be able to identify and describe 10 of his personal habits.

Note: Aids, paraprofessionals, or peer assistants may be utilized to provide help for students who have either reading or writing difficulties.

Directions: (Teacher)

1. Duplicate "Habits I Have" chart (see p. 221).

Suggested Follow-Ups:

1. In small groups, let students share some of the *harmful* habits they have listed and indicate to the others in the group:
   a. all of the information on the chart related to these harmful habits,
   b. whether he/she believes this habit is harmful to others as well as to himself/herself, and
   c. how he/she might go about changing this habit.
2. List as many reasons as students can think of why habits are so difficult to break.
3. Agree on one answer to the stem sentence: "Smoking becomes a habit that . . ."

What Can I Do?[16]

Concept:

The use of substances that modify mood and behavior arises from a variety of motivations.

[16] Developed by Nick Alexandrou, Lacy Harless, Cheryl Holloway, Florence Mazzaferro, Tallmadge (Ohio) City Schools.

HABITS I HAVE

Directions: Fill out chart as completely as possible.

List 10 Habits here	I think I started this habit because	Things that happened because I have this habit	Does this habit help me or harm me?
1. Example: Biting my fingernails	I was bored	I get yelled at. My fingers are ugly.	Harm
2.			
3.			
4.			
5.			
6.			
7.			
8.			
9.			
10.			

General Behavioral Objective:

The students will be able to identify alternative behaviors to the use of mood and/or behavior modifying substances.

Domain: Affective   *Dimension:* Social

Grade Level: Upper elementary

Specific Behavioral Objective:

In small groups, the students will be able to list the possible behaviors to a situation involving either cigarettes or pills.

Directions: (Teacher)

1. Duplicate "What Can I Do" worksheet (see p. 222).
2. Organize class into groups of 4-6.

221

Suggested Follow-Ups:

1. Individually rank the behaviors that were listed by the group, from "The one I would least likely do" (#1) to "The one I would most likely do" (# ?).

2. After the students have completed their rankings, explain that all behaviors have results (consequences) and that a behavior is usually judged "good" or "bad" by the way it affects either the individual or other people.

"WHAT CAN I DO?"
WORKSHEET

Directions:

1. Group is to choose *one* of the following situations. Circle the number.

2. List all of the ways to behave that your group can think of.

Situation 1:

You are playing outside with a small group of your friends. One of your friends takes a bag from his pocket containing several brightly colored objects. He says, "I took these from my big brother's secret hiding place. I heard him tell one of his friends that they really make you feel good. How about trying one?"

Situation 2:

You are walking home from school with three friends. One of them says, "Hey, I swiped a package of cigarettes from my mom. Let's take them over to the park and smoke them."

List of Behaviors:

1.
2.
3.
4.
5.
6.
7.
8.
9.
10.

Should I? Shouldn't I?

Concept:

The use of substances that modify mood and behavior arises from a variety of motivations.

General Behavioral Objective:

The student will be able to evaluate the forces that influence people to use or not use substances that modify mood or behavior.

Domain: Affective   *Dimension:* Social

Grade Level: Upper elementary

Specific Behavioral Objective:

After observing a role-playing situation involving medication offered by a friend, the student will be able to identify the social forces that influence people by completing an observation guide.

Directions: (Teacher)

1. Duplicate "Should I? Shouldn't I?" Observation Guide (see p. 224).
2. Choose the three participants. Give each one of the role descriptions.
3. Brief the remainder of class as observers.
4. Read the situation to entire class.
5. Stop the action when Role Player "B" makes a decision.

Suggested Follow-Up:

1. Discuss the answers to the questions on the observation guide.
2. Other discussion questions:
   a. In your opinion why was the decision "B" made wise or unwise?
   b. What are the possible results (consequences) if the decision is to take the pill? if the decision is not to take the pill?
   c. What commonly-used substance might the pills have been?

"Should I? Shouldn't I?"

SITUATION AND ROLE DESCRIPTIONS[17]

Situation:

You and your friend are playing at your house and he/she becomes ill. Your brother/sister, who is one year older, is at home too. Your

[17] Situation developed by Joanne Smith, Barbara Watral, Jan Karl, Janelle Falcone, Tallmadge (Ohio) City Schools.

mother is not at home so you say, "Mom always gives me pills when I get sick. I'll go get you some from the medicine cabinet."

Roles:

Role A. You are ten years old. You are the person who gets the pills for your friend. Try to talk him/her into taking the pills. Use all the reasons you can think of why your friend should take the pills. You feel important because you are helping your friend.

Role B. You are ten years old. You are the person who is ill. You are not sure whether you should take the medicine your friend offers you or not. You are to ask many questions about it to give you time to make up your mind. Ask such questions as, "Does it taste bad?" and "What is it?" and "Are you sure it's O.K. to take it?" You decide whether you want to take the pill or not. You don't know whether to listen to your friend or to his/her brother/sister.

Role C. You are eleven years old. You hear your brother/sister offer his/her friend some pills. You question whether it's OK or not. You say, "Maybe you should go home and tell your mother that you are sick" or "Why don't you wait 'till mom gets home?" or "How do you know it won't make him/her worse?"

OBSERVATION GUIDE

1. What reasons are used to get the person to take the pill?

2. What reasons are used to keep the person from taking the pill?

3. What swayed the person to make the decision that he/she did?

4. What would cause you to decide . . .
   a. to take the pill?

   b. not to take the pill?

"What Will Happen If . . .?"

SITUATION AND ROLE DESCRIPTION[18]

Situation:

Three friends are in the school lunch room. When they sit down at the table with their lunch, they find a capsule (KAP-sul) on the table.

Roles:

Role A. You want to give the capsule to the principal. Try to get the others to agree. Say things like, "We don't know what it is," or "It might hurt someone."

Role B. You want the other kids to think you are cool. You are the class show-off. Try to get one of your friends to take the capsule. If that doesn't work, then say, "If you're that chicken, I'll take it myself."

Role C. You want to be the center of attention. You are always playing jokes on other people. You want to put the capsule in someone else's milk. Try to get your friends to agree with you.

Concept:

The use of substances that modify mood and behavior arises from a variety of motivations.

General Behavioral Objective:

The student will be able to evaluate the forces that influence people to use or not use substances that modify mood or behavior.

Domain: Affective   *Dimension:* Social, Physical

Grade Level: Upper elementary

---

[18] Situation developed by Pauline Harless, Jean Shaw, Richard Johnson, Tallmadge (Ohio) City Schools.

Specific Behavioral Objective 1:

After observing a role playing situation, the student will be able to identify verbally the possible social and physical consequences of choosing to use or not use an unknown substance.

Directions: (Teacher)

1. Select three students of the same sex for the role play.
2. Provide role descriptions for the participants (see p. 225).
3. Brief the observers: While you are watching the role play:
    a. Decide how each person might be treated by friends, by teachers or principal, or by parents if he/she were to DO what he/she suggests to the others.
    b. Decide what the physical results might be if the group decides to go along with either character "B" or "C."
4. Stop the action when a decision is reached.
5. Using either the chalkboard or a prepared transparency, list the possible social consequences:
    a. If the capsule is given to the principal:
        1. how friends might react
        2. how teachers or the principal might react
        3. how parents might react
    b. If the capsule is taken by one of the role players:
        1. how friends might react
        2. how teachers or the principal might react
        3. how parents might react
    c. If the capsule is put in someone else's milk:
        1. how friends might react
        2. how teachers or the principal might react
        3. how parents might react
6. Go over the list and have the students rate each item as "good news", "bad news", or "either."
7. Repeat listing the possible physical consequences for each action.

Domain: Psychomotor   *Dimension:* Social

Specific Behavioral Objective 2:

After observing the role play, the student is able to write and read a news bulletin that describes the situation.

Situation: (Student)

You are TV newscasters. Your boss has asked you to write a special news bulletin to be read on the air as soon as possible concerning the role playing situation.

   1. You may work alone or in dyads.

   2. Each news bulletin should include:

     a. *who* was involved

     b. *how* the event occurred

     c. *where* it occurred

     d. *what* the results (consequences) of the behavior were

   3. Record your bulletin on the cassette.

Domain: Affective   *Dimension:* Emotional

Specific Behavioral Objective 3:

Using the role play behaviors, the student is able to select a personal behavior by values voting.

Directions: (Teacher)

   1. On 5″ × 8″ cards or white poster paper, print the phrases:

     a. WOULD REPORT IT TO THE PRINCIPAL

     b. WOULD TAKE CAPSULE MYSELF

     c. WOULD TRY TO GET SOMEONE ELSE TO TAKE IT

     d. WOULD PUT IN SOMEONE'S MILK

     e. NONE OF THE OTHER CHOICES

   2. Place the printed phrases on the floor at scattered positions.

Directions: (Student)

   1. Move to the position that best describes what you think your behavior would be if you were in this situation.

Suggested Follow-Up:

   1. Discussion:

     a. If you select "None of the other choices," what would you do?

     b. What are your reasons for making the choice that you did?

Little People Power Campaign

Concept:

The use of substances that modify mood and behavior arises from a variety of motivations.

General Behavioral Objective:

The students will be able to identify alternate behaviors to the use of mood and/or behavior modifying substances.

Domain: Psychomotor   *Dimension:* Social

Grade Level: Upper elementary

Specific Behavioral Objective:

In small groups, the students will be able to prepare one portion of an advertising campaign presenting alternative behaviors to the use of tobacco.

Situation:

The members of this class are all employees of the advertising firm "Little People Power." Your company has been hired to sell parents on the idea of choosing other things to do instead of smoking.

Directions: (Teacher)

    1. Provide materials needed for the projects.
    2. Designate areas for each group.

Directions: (Students)

1. Each group of three or four is a team.
2. Each team choose one activity.
   a. As an art project, draw a picture to give to a smoker in your family with the caption: "Instead of Smoking Why Not Do This With Me? Or with Mom? Or with Dad?"
   b. Plan a skit for the PTA entitled: "Instead of Smoking, You'll Enjoy . . . "
   c. Write the words to a song, "Try It, You'll Like It". Choose a tune everyone in group knows. After rehearsing the song, record it on a cassette.
   d. Make up slogans for use on picket signs for open house or PTA meeting.
   e. Write a short speech to give in other rooms. Explain the "Little People Power" campaign. The purpose of the

speech is to influence other students to talk to parents who smoke and to suggest other things they could do instead of smoking.

Suggested Follow-Ups:

1. Have a total school "Little People Power" campaign with students in this class spearheading the drive.
2. Present the entire program to the parents at a PTA program.
3. Display art projects in hallways.
4. Use similiar theme for other concepts.

---

concept 10:

Food Selection and Eating Patterns Are Determined by Physical, Social, Mental, Economic and Cultural Factors

---

Introduction to Concept — Lower Elementary Level

TILLIE THE TEMPTRESS

Tillie the Temptress is not a real person. You can't see her at all. But you can believe that she is with you, and everyone else, all of the time. Every now and then she pops up and whispers in your head trying to get you to do, say, or think things you know you really shouldn't. Sometimes you give in to her and do the things *she* wants you to do. Other times you are strong and you do the things *you* know are best.

One of the ways Tillie the Temptress tries to run your life is by telling you *how* you should eat, *what* you should eat, and *when* you should eat. Have you ever felt her telling you such things as:

"Put sugar on it to make it taste better"?

"Eat only the things you like"?

"Don't try anything new — you may not like it"?

"Don't bother to chew your food — just swallow it when you are in a hurry"?

"Skip the vegetables! If you get hungry later, there's always candy and chips"?

"Drink soda pop between and with meals — it's so refreshing"?

"Eat what you like before meals! You may not like what is being served"?

"Forget breakfast — it's a drag"?

"Use your lunch money to buy snacks on the way home from school.'"?

Can you think of some other things Tillie the Temptress tries to tell you that might keep you from eating right?

Do you give in to Tillie most of the time, or are you strong most of the time?

You now know that Tillie the Temptress is the name we have given to the character that tries to get you to do the things that aren't good for you. Can you think of a good name for the character that helps you to be strong enough to do the right things and sometimes win the battle with Tillie?

Can you draw a picture of Tillie the Temptress and (your other character) fighting over your eating habits?

Foods in Groups

Concept:

Food selection and eating patterns are determined by physical, social, mental, economic, and cultural factors.

General Behavioral Objective:

The student will be able to identify foods that belong in the Basic Four food groups.

Domain: Cognitive   *Dimension:* Mental

Grade Level: Lower elementary

Specific Behavioral Objective:

Using food model cards, the student is able to identify the food groups to which they belong by placing them on the chalkboard diagram.

Directions: (Teacher)

1. Construct a diagram of five columns on the chalkboard using magnetic tape, masking tape, or chalk.
2. Head the columns: Grain, Fruit-Vegetable, Milk, Meat, Others.
3. Prepare the food model cards by attaching small pieces of magnetic tape to the back or put loops of masking tape in the board columns.
4. Put food model cards in large grocery sacks. Eliminate cards that are combinations of two groups (sandwiches).

Directions: (Student)

1. Draw two food model cards from the sack.

2. All students who have foods in the fruit and vegetable group put them on the chalkboard in the proper column.

3. The class evaluates the correctness of the placement.

4. Repeat with each food group.

Suggested Follow-Up:

1. Using the food model cards on the chalkboard, have individual students select foods that they would like to eat for (a) breakfast, (b) lunch, and (c) dinner. Tell them that they must have foods from each of the Basic Four food groups in each meal.

Suggested Teaching Aid:

Food Model Packet, National Dairy Council.

Where Does It Grow?

Concept:

Food selection and eating patterns are determined by physical, social, mental, economic, and cultural factors.

General Behavioral Objective:

The student will be able to identify the source of foods.

Domain: Cognitive   *Dimension:* Mental

Grade Level: Lower elementary

Specific Behavioral Objective:

Using food model cards, the student is able to identify plant products that grow above the ground and those that grow in the ground by placing them on a chalkboard diagram.

Directions: (Teacher)

1. Put a strip of magnetic tape across the chalkboard.
2. Label the upper portion "Above Ground" and the lower section "In the Ground."
3. Put food model cards from plant sources in a box.

Directions: (Student)

1. Choose one picture from the box.
2. If your fruit or vegetable grows above the ground, place it above the line; if it grows in the ground, place it below the line.

Suggested Follow-Ups:

1. Name the fruit or vegetable.
2. Tell whether it grows on a plant, a bush or a tree.

Animal, Fish or Fowl

Concept:

Food selection and eating patterns are determined by physical, social, mental, economic, and cultural factors.

General Behavioral Objective:

The student will be able to identify the source of foods.

Domain: Cognitive   *Dimension:* Mental

Grade Level: Lower elementary

Specific Behavioral Objective:

Using flash cards, the student is able to identify the source of meat and dairy products by moving to the correct area of the room.

Directions: (Teacher)

1. Dry mount pictures of meat and dairy products on construction paper or tag board for the "Players."
2. Print the appropriate label on each.
3. For the "Leaders," prepare cards for "cow," "pig," "sheep," "poultry," and "fish/shellfish."
4. Give the "Leader" cards to five students. Direct each to an area of the room.
5. Pass out one "Player" card to each student.

Directions: (Student)

1. Move to the animal, fowl, or fish that is the source of your product.

Pig	Cow	Sheep
Ham	Milk	Lamb chop
Bacon	Butter	Leg of lamb
Pork chop	Veal chop	Roast lamb
Pork liver	Hamburger	
Pork roast	Swiss steak	
Canadian bacon	T-bone steak	
Spare ribs	Beef liver	
Sausage	Beef heart	
	Tongue	
	Tripe	

Poultry	Fish/Shellfish
Eggs	Smoked salmon
Fried chicken	Creamed cod fish
Roast duck	Lobster tails
Giblets	Hard shell crabs
Roast goose	Oyster stew
Turkey pot pie	Fried clams
	Shrimp cocktail

Alternative Suggestions:

1. Use cards as flash cards. The student who identifies the source first gets the card.
2. Divide the cards into two groups. Divide the class into two teams with each participant having a card.
   a. Player A-1 shows card to player B-1.
   b. Team B receives 2 points for two correct answers (product and source) and 1 point for either product or source.
   c. Team A receives 2 points if no correct answer is given.
   d. Player from Team B shows the next card.

What Food Am I?

Concept:

Food selection and eating patterns are determined by physical, social, mental, economic, and cultural factors.

General Behavioral Objective:

The student will be able to describe different foods.

Domain: Cognitive   *Dimension:* Physical

Grade Level: Lower elementary

Specific Behavioral Objective:

Using selected food model cards, the student will be able to present verbal and nonverbal clues describing the physical properties of a specific food for the class to identify.

Directions: (Student)

1. Choose any two foods from the food model cards and take them back to your seat so that no one else can see them. Do not tell *anyone* what your foods are.
2. When your turn comes, tell the class about one of the foods you have chosen by saying:
   a. I am a food.
   b. I belong to the _____ food group (tell if you belong to the fruit and vegetable group, the milk group, the meat group, or the bread and cereal group).
   c. I am . . . (tell the color(s) you are).
   d. My name begins with the letter _____.

3. If you wish you may then act out without words what you look like.
4. When you have finished ask the class, "What food am I?" and let them guess.
5. The person who guesses correctly becomes the "Leader."

Suggested Teaching Aids:

Food Model Packet, National Dairy Council.

Foods for Special Occasions

Concept:

Food selection and eating patterns are determined by physical, social, mental, economic, and cultural patterns.

General Behavioral Objective:

The student will be able to cite occasions when special foods are eaten.

Domain: Psychomotor   *Dimension:* Social

Grade Level: Lower elementary

Specific Behavioral Objectives:

1. From a list of special occasions, the student will be able to draw a picture of the event.
2. Using magazine pictures of food, the student will be able to illustrate favorite foods for the selected occasion by mounting the pictures on the drawing.

Directions: (Teacher)

1. Print each of the following special occasions on pieces of tagboard ahead of time.

FOURTH OF JULY PICNIC	VISITING GRANDMOTHER
ICE SKATING OR SWIMMING PARTY	CHRISTMAS
MY BIRTHDAY	EASTER
CAMPING OUT	ROSH HASHANA (ha-SHAH-nah)
YOM KIPPUR (yom-kih-POOR)	FAMILY REUNION (ree-YOU-yun)
EATING AT A RESTAURANT	VACATION
(RES-toe-rahnt)	VALENTINE PARTY
HALLOWEEN PARTY	

2. Have students suggest any other very special times that their family or friends spend together. These can be put on cards as well.

3. Place these cards on the bulletin board around the room or on the chalkboard with magnetic tape.

4. Familiarize students with new words and pronunciation.

5. Have poster size paper, crayons, scissors, paste or glue sticks, and old magazines with colored pictures of foods on a table. (Students may want to cut out pictures at home or bring in additional magazines from home).

Introduction:

Many of us like to eat special foods on special occasions. It's part of the fun of doing things with others. Some of these special occasions have been placed on cards around the room. Let's read these together and see if we can pronounce them.

Directions: (Student)

1. From this list choose one special occasion that you really enjoy.

2. Take a piece of poster paper from the table and draw a picture of your special occasion.

3. When you finish look through the magazines and find pictures of foods that you like to eat on this occasion. Cut them out.

4. Paste these pictures on the same paper with your picture. You can put them at the bottom or anywhere else on the sheet you care to.

5. When you are done find the label card for your fun occasion and hang your poster there.

Suggested Follow-Up:

1. Have students play "I'm thinking of a food . . ."
   a. Each student will select one food that is on his/her poster.
   b. Pupil will stand in front of the class and say, "I am thinking of a food that I love to eat on/when/at (this occasion).
   c. Pupils will look at his/her poster and try to guess the food. The one who guesses correctly then takes his turn. No one may answer unless he/she raises his/her hand and is chosen by the "it" student.

Food Selection and Eating Patterns are Determined
by Social, Physical, Mental, Economic, and
Cultural Factors.

Introduction to Concept — Upper Elementary Level

NEEDS AND NUTRITION

All of us have certain basic physical needs that must be met so that
we can continue living and doing all of the things we like, want, and
need to do. We need to have good air to breathe, water to drink, and
food to eat. Our bodies need exercise, rest, and protection from
extremes of heat and cold as well. These needs are called *basic*
because (1) without any one of them we would die, and (2) each
need is dependent on the others for its own existence. If we say each
need is, in itself, necessary to life then we must realize that *all needs
are important and none is more important than the others.* This is
what is meant by the phrase "*basic* needs."

In this next part of our health education we are going to be learning
more about one of these basic needs — the food we eat. Food is the
fuel we use to keep our body machine running. Can you tell me what
are some other kinds of fuels that keep other kinds of machines
running?

Meeting our nutritional needs is very important to each of us. The
foods we choose to eat and the eating habits that each of us develop
over the years determine how well our body machine works and how
long it will run. Having enough food is important, but having enough
of the right foods is even more important. The right foods are nutritional foods — those that provide what the body requires to function properly.

In this concept we will be doing some activities that will assist us in
LEARNING about food and nutrition, check out *FEELINGS* about

the food we eat, and decide what we can be *DOING* to help ourselves and others meet our nutritional needs.

Foods I Like

Concept:

Food selection and eating patterns are determined by physical, social, economic, mental, and cultural factors.

General Behavioral Objective:

The student will be able to explain personal likes and dislikes of foods.

Domain: Affective   *Dimension:* Social

Grade Level: Upper elementary

Specific Behavioral Objective:

By completing a series of stem sentences, the student will be able to identify the foods personally preferred in different social situations.

Introduction: (Student)

We all like some foods better than others. Not everyone likes the same things. If we are with friends we may prefer different foods than we would if we were with our family. Or our choices can change if it's a special occasion, such as a birthday, a holiday, a picnic, or eating in a restaurant. This activity will help you identify the foods you like the best in different situations.

1. On my birthday Mom says I can have four friends over for dinner and I can choose the food. I think I will select this menu . . .

2. My favorite holiday is . . .; we always celebrate by having special foods such as . . .

3. When our family eats at a restaurant, I usually order . . .

4. At a picnic my favorite food is . . .

5. If I could have only *one* thing for a snack, I would choose to have . . .

6. For breakfast, my favorite drink is . . .; for dinner, my favorite drink is . . .

7. If I drink something between meals, it is usually . . .

8. The dessert I like the most after a meal is . . .

Suggested Follow-Up:

1. Class discussion:
   a. the different foods selected
   b. why the foods are liked

Identifying Nutrients

Concept:

Food selection and eating patterns are determined by physical, social, mental, economic, and cultural patterns.

General Behavioral Objective:

The student will be able to identify nutrients and some foods that supply each.

Domain: Cognitive   *Dimension:* Physical

Grade Level: Upper elementary

Specific Behavioral Objective:

When given a series of food pictures, the student will be able to identify the nutrients found in each by drawing a line from the food to the nutrients.

Directions: (Teacher)

1. Duplicate the worksheet on p. 240.
2. Define the term "nutrients."
3. Read the directions to the class.

Directions: (Student)

1. All of the food pictures on the left side of the worksheet contain nutrients (NEW-tree-unts).
2. Using the resource materials available on the table, find out which nutrients are present in each food.

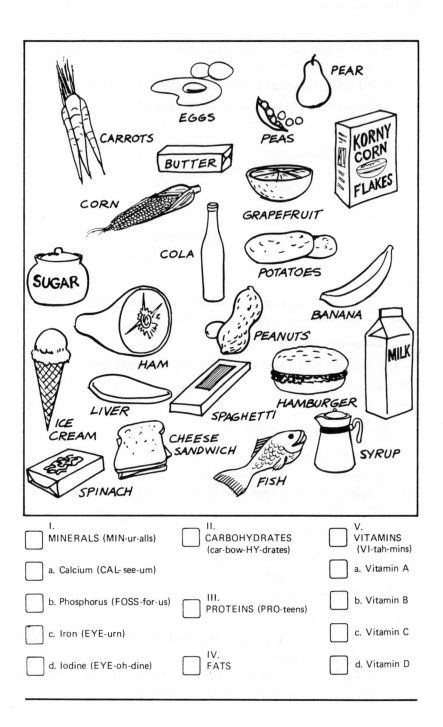

CARROTS

EGGS

PEAR

PEAS

BUTTER

KORNY CORN FLAKES

CORN

GRAPEFRUIT

COLA

SUGAR

POTATOES

BANANA

HAM

PEANUTS

MILK

ICE CREAM

LIVER

SPAGHETTI

HAMBURGER

SPINACH

CHEESE SANDWICH

FISH

SYRUP

I.
MINERALS (MIN-ur-alls)

a. Calcium (CAL- see-um)

b. Phosphorus (FOSS-for-us)

c. Iron (EYE-urn)

d. Iodine (EYE-oh-dine)

II.
CARBOHYDRATES
(car-bow-HY-drates)

III.
PROTEINS (PRO-teens)

IV.
FATS

V.
VITAMINS
(VI-tah-mins)

a. Vitamin A

b. Vitamin B

c. Vitamin C

d. Vitamin D

3. Draw a line from the food to each block of a nutrient which is in that food.

4. There may be one or more than one nutrient in each food.

Suggested Follow-Up:

Place food model pictures on a table in four sections according to food groups spread out as in a cafeteria line. Students pass through the line and select foods that they would prefer for a particular meal. By looking on the back of each food picture, read and list the nutrients found in all of the foods in their meal. Keep score each time a nutrient is present. Answer the following questions:

1. In the meal I selected which nutrient(s) was/were present in the greatest number?

2. Which nutrient(s) was/were not in any of the foods I selected?

3. If I wanted to have each nutrient represented, I would probably have to substitute some other foods for some that I chose. What substitutions could I make?

Guess the Food

Concept:

Food selection and eating patterns are determined by physical, social, mental, economic, and cultural patterns.

General Behavioral Objective:

The student will be able to describe different foods.

Domain: Cognitive   *Dimension:* Physical

Grade Level: Upper elementary

Specific Behavioral Objective:

Using a selected food comparison card, the student will be able to describe the component parts and qualities of a food of his choice by presenting verbal clues.

Directions: (Student)

1. The food comparison cards are face down on the front table. Choose one without looking at it and take it back to your seat. *Be sure that no one else sees it.*

2. On a small piece of paper jot down the information about (1) which food group this food belongs to, (2) what nutrients (and in what amount) are found in this food, and (3) how many calories there are in a certain size serving.

3. When your turn comes, share this information verbally with the class. Start out by saying:

   a. "I am a food."

   b. "I am a member of the _____ food group."

   c. "In a _____ oz./mg. serving of me, I will provide your body with _____ calories."

   d. "I am made up of these nutrients." (Give the nutrients starting with those in the largest amount).

   e. "What food am I?"

4. The person answering correctly takes your place. In case the person answering has already had a turn, he/she chooses someone else.

5. If no one guesses correctly from the information you have given, you may want to act out without using words (charade) what this food looks like, sounds like, or comes from.

Suggested Teaching Aids:

Food Comparison Cards, National Dairy Council.

What Would I Do?

Concept:

Food selection and eating patterns are determined by physical, social, economic, mental, and cultural factors.

General Behavioral Objective:

The student will be able to apply the behavioral equation to his own food selection and eating patterns.

Domain: Affective   *Dimension:* Emotional

Grade Level: Upper elementary

Specific Beahvioral Objectives:

1. When given a situation involving not being hungry, the student is able, on a given activity sheet, to generate possible reasons for the condition, to choose possible personal behaviors, and to predict the probable consequences.

2. After completing the above, the student is able to select the behavior and consequences he would prefer.

Directions: (Teacher)

1. Dupplicate the "What Would I Do?" worksheet (see p. 244).

Directions: (Student)

1. Use the activity sheet provided.
2. Read the situation.
3. Follow the directions and fill out the chart.

Suggested Follow-Ups:

1. Share preferences in class discussion.
2. Write their preferred behavior and consequence on the board. If it is the same as someone else's, do not repeat.
3. From those now listed on the board, individually rank all behaviors from those that he/she most prefers to the one he/she least prefers.
4. Make up a newspaper headline concerning his/her behavior and consequence preference. For example:
   JIM SMITH TELLS MOM HE DOESN'T FEEL LIKE EATING; SHE FAINTS!

"WHAT WOULD I DO?" WORKSHEET

Situation:

Your mother calls, "Dinner is ready!" You don't feel like eating.

Directions:

Fill out the chart below. For each reason you give, be sure to have a behavior and at least *one* possible consequence.

Reasons	Behavior	Consequences
I might not be hungry because . . .	Therefore, I would . . .	If I behaved this way my Mom/Dad/others would probably . . .

1	1	1
2	2	2
3	3	3
4	4	4

Of the behaviors listed and the resulting consequence, the one I would prefer is . . .

concept 11:

Emotional Health is Influenced by Interpersonal Relationships and Enhanced by an Understanding of the Factors Affecting Behavior.

Introduction To Concept — Lower Elementary Level
FREDDY THE FRIENDLY BEAR CUB

Freddy the Friendly Bear Cub is sitting over in the corner crying. What do you suppose has happened that is making him cry?

What has really happened is that Freddy's family has just moved

244

from where they used to live far away on the other side of the forest. Back there Freddy was very happy. He had many playmates, and together they would run and play and wrestle among the leaves that had fallen to the ground. When he was a tiny bear, Freddy had tumbled out of a tree and hurt his front leg. It caused him to limp, and he couldn't run as fast as the others. But his friends didn't care because they liked Freddy. He was friendly and fun.

One day Freddy's father came home and announced to his family that they were going to have to move far away to the other side of the forest. Freddy was sorry to leave his friends, but he understood that his family had no choice.

When they reached their new home, Freddy felt a little better because he saw that there were many other cubs about his age, and he began to think how nice it would be to run and play and wrestle among the fallen leaves with his new friends.

After they got settled in their new home, Freddy ran out to find the cubs he had seen playing when he first arrived. There they were over across the patch of bushes! When they saw him running to join them, they stopped playing and stared at him.

Jimmy Cub called out, "Who are you and what are you doing here?"

Kathy Cub said, "You don't belong here!"

Scotty Cub cried out, "We don't like to let strange cubs play with us."

Terry Cub turned to the others and said, "Look how funny he walks and runs. We don't want to play with him." And they started to run and play and wrestle among the leaves once again.

Freddy backed away with his head hanging very low. Before he knew it, huge tears were escaping from his warm, brown eyes.

Jimmy Cub's mother happened to be walking by and spotted Freddy over in a corner of the grassy play area. When she got closer she could see his tears glistening in the sunshine. She walked over and in a very kind voice asked him why he was crying. Freddy told her what had happened. Jimmy's mother explained to Freddy that most cubs don't understand that all bears, cubs or grown-ups, need to be liked by other bears and to be included in their groups whether they are playing or working. She told Freddy to follow her, and together they walked over and joined the playful cubs. Jimmy's mother introduced Freddy to each and every one of them. She explained that Freddy had just moved to their part of the woods, and she also told them how Freddy hurt his leg when he was a tiny cub. When Jimmy's mother finished talking, Kathy Cub asked Freddy if he would like to play with them. Freddy answered, "Oh, yes!"

It wasn't long before he was running and playing and wrestling among the fallen leaves with his new friends. And Freddy was showing them that, even though he couldn't run as fast as they could, he was friendly and fun. Freddy was very happy that the others had accepted him, and he felt that they would grow to like one another very much.

We are going to be learning about our inner feelings (emotions) and doing many things to help us to learn. Don't you think it would be fun if some of you would act out the story I have just read to you?

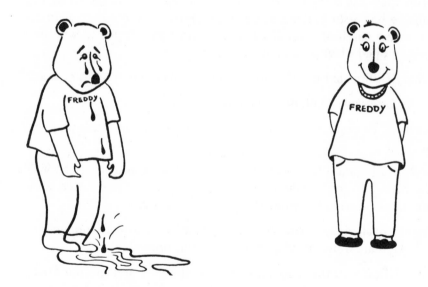

Freddy the Friendly Bear Cub Skit

Concept:

Emotional health is influenced by interpersonal relationships and enhanced by an understanding of the factors affecting behavior.

General Behavioral Objective:

The student will be able to cite the relationship between needs, feelings, and behavior.

Domain: Psychomotor   *Dimension:* Mental, Emotional

Grade Level: Lower elementary

Specific Behavioral Objective:

After listening to the story of Freddy the Friendly Bear Cub, the students will be able to portray the needs and feelings by acting out the story.

Directions:

1. The teacher will assign students the following parts in the story (parts may be interchanged):
   a. Freddy the Friendly Bear Cub (or Frances the Friendly Bear Cub)
   b. Freddy's mother
   c. Freddy's father
   d. Freddy's playmates at his former home
   e. Jimmy Cub
   f. Kathy Cub
   g. Scotty Cub
   h. Terry Cub
   i. The other cubs at Freddy's new home
   j. Jimmy Cub's mother
2. The scenes:
   a. Freddy playing with his friends in the forest
   b. At home
   c. At Freddy's new home
   d. Out in the forest with the cubs

Suggested Follow-Up Discussion:

1. Jimmy Cub's mother said that all bears, big or small, need what two things?
2. Is this true for all people as well?
3. What kinds of *feelings* did Freddy have in this story?
4. Our inner feelings are called our emotions. Freddy's emotions were *sadness* and *happiness*. How might we know if Freddy is happy or sad? Can you tell me some other inner feelings that *people* have?
5. Do people need the same two things that Jimmy Cub's mother said all bears need?

6. Can we change the story around and put people into it instead of bears? Tell me how this might be.

Events Cause Feelings

Concept:

Emotional health is influenced by interpersonal relationships and enhanced by an understanding of the factors affecting behavior.

General Behavioral Objective:

The student is able to cite the relationship between emotions and behavior.

Domain: Affective   *Dimension:* Mental, Emotional

Grade Level: Lower elementary

Specific Behavioral Objective:

When given a series of stem sentences, the student is able to describe the events that cause him to feel a specific emotion.

Directions: (Teacher)

1. If students can read and write, duplicate the "Events Cause Feelings" worksheet (see p. 249).
2. If students are nonreaders, read the stem sentences for them to respond verbally.

Introduction:

Some of us are *like* many other people in the world in many ways. What are some of these ways? Some of us are *different* from many other people in many ways. Can you tell me some of the ways we are different?

One of the things we share with all other people is that we have inner feelings that are called emotions. Let's make a list of these inner feelings on the board. Sometimes we just keep these feelings inside. Sometimes we feel so strongly that we do something to show others how we feel. For example, when we are very sad or very hurt, we cry. Can you tell some other ways we show our strong feelings?

There is always something that happens (an event) before we feel anything inside. This is something that *causes* us to feel the way we do. For example: "When my pet gerbil died, I felt very sad and I cried." Can you tell me what the *event* in this example is? What is the *feeling word*? How did I *behave* (what did I *do*) to show that I felt this way? There is always something that causes us to feel the way we do, and something that happens because we feel that way.

Suggested Follow-Ups:

1. Sharing of answers should be *voluntary*.
2. Students may share and compare their answers with those of their classmates by any one of the following techniques:
   a. Small group discussions in which members answer questions such as:
      1. When was the last time you got very, very angry?
      2. What scares you the most?
      3. Have you ever been jealous? Of what?
      4. When do you feel loved the most?
   b. Each child writing his response to *one* of the sentences on the blackboard.
   c. General class discussion answering questions such as those stated above or taking turns reading or telling responses to stem sentences.
   d. Show class a "Love is . . ." or "Happiness is . . ." cartoon. Have student draw a cartoon in either of the two categories expressing his feelings as to what *love* or *happiness* is.

"EVENTS CAUSE FEELINGS" WORKSHEET

Directions:

Finish each of these stem sentences by giving an event that makes you feel the emotion given. There is no right or wrong answer.

1. I feel happy when . . .
2. I get angry when . . .
3. I enjoy . . .
4. I don't like to . . .
5. I am afraid when . . .
6. I feel brave when . . .
7. I am bothered if . . .
8. I feel uneasy if . . .
9. I laugh whenever . . .
10. I am embarrassed if I . . .
11. I am sad when . . .
12. I am disappointed when . . .
13. I feel jealous when . . .
14. I feel excited when . . .
15. I get butterflies in my stomach when . . .

Emotions and Events

Concept:

Emotional health is influenced by interpersonal relationships and enhanced by an understanding of the factors affecting behavior.

General Behavioral Objective:

The student is able to cite the relationship between emotions and behavior.

Domain: Cognitive   *Dimension:* Mental, Emotional

Grade Level: Lower elementary

Specific Behavioral Objective:

Using the completed "Events Cause Feelings" Worksheet, the student is able to identify the emotion and the behavior or event in each sentence by listing them on an activity sheet.

Directions: (Teacher)

1. Duplicate the "Emotion and Events" worksheet. (see p. 251).

Suggested Follow-Up:

1. Transparency
    a. Draw the activity sheet format without numbers on an acetate. Use an overhead projector.
    b. Go through the sentences recording the "feeling" word from the sentence and list all of the behaviors or events given verbally by the students.
2. Flash Cards
    a. Make flash cards of each emotion with its phonetic pronunciation.
        1. Pronounce the word.
        2. Use it correctly in a sentence.
    b. Make flash cards of the behaviors or events.
        1. Verbalize emotions generated by each.
    c. Put magnetic tape on all flash cards.
        1. Place on chalkboard randomly.

250

2. Identify emotions vs. behaviors/events by moving cards to proper columns.

3. Using selected behaviors, match as many emotions as can be justified. Example: "Yelling at me" — anger, fear, embarrassment.

d. Include new words in spelling lesson.

e. Choose an emotion and write a short story:

1. telling about events leading up to the emotional response, and

2. telling what happened (consequences) as a result of the emotional response.

f. Share stories by:

1. recording on a cassette

2. using hand puppets

"EMOTIONS AND EVENTS" WORKSHEET

Directions:

1. Pick out the "feeling" word or emotion (ee-MO-shun) in each of the sentences. Write the words in Column 1.

2. Pick out the "behavior" (act) or the event in each sentence that makes you feel the emotion. Write the behaviors or events in Column 2.

Column 1	*Column 2*
Feeling word (emotion)	Behavior or event
1.	1.
2.	2.
3.	3.
4.	4.
5.	5.
6.	6.
7.	7.
8.	8.
9.	9.
10.	10.
11.	11.
12.	12.
13.	13.
14.	14.
15.	15.

I Feel . . .

Concept:

Emotional health is influenced by interpersonal relationships and enhanced by an understanding of the factors affecting behavior.

General Behavioral Objective:

The student is able to cite the relationship between emotions and behavior.

Domain: Affective   *Dimension:* Mental, Emotional

Grade Level: Lower elementary

Specific Behavioral Objective:

When a series of situations is read, the student is able to show how each makes him/her feel by circling one of four cartoon faces depicting the emotions.

Directions: (Teacher)

1. Duplicate the worksheet on p. 253.

Directions: (Student)

Circle the face that best tells how you would feel when these things happen:

1. When someone calls me a bad name, I feel . . .
2. When I hear strange noises in the night, I feel . . .
3. When my puppy sits in my lap, I feel . . .
4. When I hear one of my classmates is sick, I feel . . .
5. When I watch a monster movie on TV, I feel . . .

Suggested Follow-Up:

1. Class discussion:
   a. Think of the times when you have been happy — sad — angry — afraid.
   b. Describe (tell us) what happened that made you feel that way.
2. Role play:
   a. Use the situations brought out in the class discussions.
   b. Show how you *act* when you are happy — sad — angry — afraid.
   c. Since not everyone *acts* the same way, who can show us how he/she acts that is different?

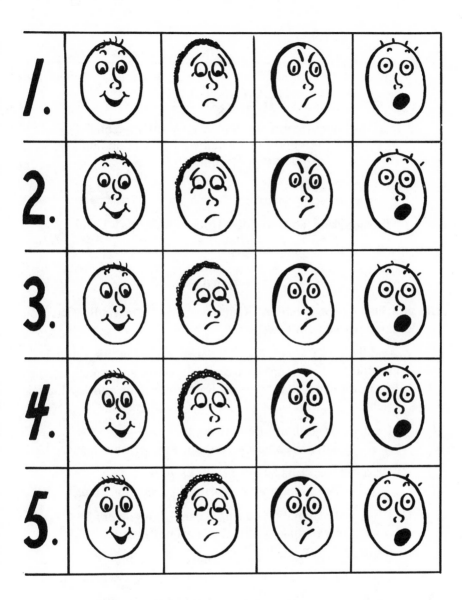

3. Drawing:

  a. Choose one of the "feelings."

  b. Draw a picture of one thing that makes you feel the happiest, the saddest, the angriest, or the most afraid.

  c. Show the picture to the class and tell about it.

Emotional Health is Influenced by Interpersonal Relationships and Enhanced by an Understanding of Factors Affecting Behavior.

Introduction To Concept — Upper Elementary Level

THE RIDDLE

Do you like to solve riddles? Can you think of a riddle that you would like to share with the class?

I have a riddle. Let's see if you can figure out what this riddle is. If you think you know the answer write it down on your small piece of paper, but don't show it to anyone. Raise your hand and I will see if you are right.

CLUE 1 — Of each of you I am a part.
I live deep inside you, but I'm not your heart.

CLUE 2 — I can't be heard, I can't be seen,
But I am more powerful than any machine.

CLUE 3 — I can make you sing, I can make you cry,
I can make you quit, or even make you try.

CLUE 4 — I am behind you whenever you fight,
I make you run when you see a scary sight.

CLUE 5 — You show me to all, day in and day out,
Whether with a smile or with a huge pout.

CLUE 6 — I have no size, I have no weight.
But *all* of your actions I can regulate.

CLUE 7 — Your parents show me when they kiss you good-night.

Or even when you do something that gets them uptight.

CLUE 8 — There are eight letters in my name, don't you see?
Can you guess if I tell you I begin with an "E"?

CLUE 9 — "Feelings" is a word that means just the same,
As all of the letters that make up my name.

CLUE 10 — Anger, fear, love, jealousy, and hate,
Are just five of the many that make me so great.

CLUE 11 — If you're still having trouble finding my name,
Unscramble these letters, then you will win the game.

E T O S N O M I

How Much Do I Fear . . .?

Concept:

Emotional health is influenced by interpersonal relationships and enhanced by an understanding of the factors affecting behavior.

General Behavioral Objective:

The student will be able to identify situations that instill fear.

Domain: Affective   *Dimension:* Emotional

Grade Level: Upper elementary

Specific Behavioral Objective:

Given a series of items, the student will be able to determine how much each is feared by placing them on a forced-choice ladder diagram.

Directions: (Teacher)

1. Prepare and distribute a 10-step forced-choice ladder (see p. 149). At the bottom of the ladder, write LEAST FEARED. At the top of the ladder, write MOST FEARED. Number each step from 1 to 10, with #1 being at the bottom.
2. Read the list of fears to the students. Give them only enough time to write each on the step of their choice. After reading each separately write the key word on the chalkboard to facilitate spelling.

Directions: (Student)

Fear is a very important emotion in everyone's life. In fact, feelings of fear are necessary for our very survival. They help us to escape from dangerous situations and keep us from being hurt or even killed.

Since everyone is different from every other person, our fears are different also. What is important is that we are able to recognize what causes us to be afraid or uncomfortable and to do something about it.

1. I am going to read you a list of fears that many people your age have. You will evaluate how you feel about each on the forced-choice ladder.

2. If the items are things you fear very little, write them in on a step somewhere near the bottom of your ladder where it says LEAST FEARED. If they are things that *really* frighten you, you will want to write them on a step near the top of the ladder where it says MOST FEARED.

3. Remember these things:

   a. You can only put one fear on each step of the ladder.

   b. You will have two minutes at the end to rearrange any of the items on the ladder you wish to.

HOW MUCH DO I FEAR . . .

1. Storms
2. Snakes
3. Spiders
4. Monster movies
5. The dark
6. Strange noises
7. Older kids (that threaten you)
8. Getting lost
9. Haunted houses
10. Death or dying

Suggested Follow-Ups:

1. Chart the fears to discover which two items are least feared and which two are most feared by students in the class.

2. Ask students to suggest other fears they might have. Use these to do an additional forced-choice ladder experience.
3. Organize students into small groups. Using the list of fears provided, discuss ways of dealing with each.

Charade-An-Emotion

Concept:

Emotional health is influenced by interpersonal relationships and enhanced by an understanding of factors affecting behavior.

General Behavioral Objective:

The student will be able to identify a variety of emotions.

Domain: Cognitive   *Dimension:* Mental, Emotional

Grade Level: Upper elementary

Specific Behavioral Objective:

By watching a series of charades, the student will be able to identify the emotions expressed by listing.

Directions: (Teacher)

1. Explain what charades are.
2. Have students identify as many emotions as they can think of. Write each on chalkboard, lettering them sequentially a, b, c, etc.
3. Assign each student a number.
4. Have each student number his paper from 1 to ____ (as many as there are students).

Directions: (Student)

1. From the list of emotions on the chalkboard, choose one that you would like to act out in charades.
2. Think of how you might do your charade so that your classmates will be able to guess which emotion you are portraying.
3. Each of you will have a turn in the order of your own number.
4. When a classmate finishes a charade, guess which of the emotions was being acted out. Look at the list on the board.

When you think you know the answer, put the *letter* of the emotion on the board next to the number on your paper.

5. There are two things you need to remember:

   a. In your charade you *cannot* use any spoken words or sounds.

   b. When you know the answer, be very quiet about it. Do not share your answer with anyone. Just write the letter of the emotion on your paper and cover your answer.

Suggested Follow-Up:

1. After every student has performed, have each stand and announce to the class the emotion he used and the letter of the emotion from the list on the chalkboard.

2. Have each student evaluate his/her own answers.

3. Discuss the activity and any possibilities of dual answers.

Mature or Immature?

Concept:

Emotional health is influenced by interpersonal relationships and enhanced by an understanding of the factors affecting behavior.

General Behavioral Objective:

The student will be able to distinguish between mature and immature behavior.

Domain: Affective   *Dimension:* Emotional

Grade Level: Upper elementary

Specific Behavioral Objective:

Given a series of situations, the student will be able to cite examples of mature and immature behavior by completing stem sentences.

Directions: (Teacher)

1. Duplicate the "Mature and Immature?" worksheet (see p. 259).

2. Read introduction to students. Make sure they understand the terms "mature behavior" and "immature behavior."

Introduction:

You tell everyone how you *really* feel by the way you act.

MATURE OR IMMATURE? WORKSHEET

Directions:

Below each situation are some stem sentences. Complete each sentence with behaviors which you think fit the situation.

Situation 1:

Terry Teaser calls me a name that I do not like.

    1. I might act *immaturely* by . . .

      If I did this, Terry would probably . . .

    2. I might act *maturely* by . . .

      If I did this, Terry might . . .

Situation 2:

Dorie Dogood gets good grades in school. She always brags to me about how the teacher lets her "get away" with everything.

    1. I might act *immaturely* by . . .

      If I did this, Dorie would probably . . .

    2. I might act *maturely* by . . .

      If I did this, Dorie might . . .

Situation 3:

Nicky Nice compliments me when I do something well.

    1. I might act *immaturely* by . . .

      If I did this, Nicky would probably . . .

    2. I might act *maturely* by . . .

      If I did this, Nicky would probably . . .

Situation 4:

Gracie Goof-off does everything but start her work when she should. When she doesn't finish on time, she starts to complain and cry.

    1. I might treat Gracie in an *immature* way by . . .

      If I did this, Gracie might . . .

    2. I would be treating Gracie *maturely* if I . . .

Situation 5:

Willie Whiner is always complaining about the way things are.

    1. I might treat Willie in an *immature* way by . . .

      If I did this, Willie would probably . . .

    2. I might treat Willie in a *mature* way by . . .

      If I did this, Willie might . . .

Sometimes you do things that are very childish. This is called *immature behavior*. When you behave immaturely, you create new problems.

Sometimes you do things that are very helpful to yourself and others. This shows that you are beginning to think things through to come up with the best answer to a problem. This is called *mature behavior*.

Mature means growing up.

Immature means remaining a child.

Suggested Follow-Ups:

    1. Discuss:
        a. Reasons for identifying the personal behaviors given as either "mature" or "immature."
        b. The variety of reactions suggested.
    2. Request students to tell of other situations in which they have reacted with either mature or immature behavior.

Sharing Feelings Is Important!

Concept:

Emotional health is influenced by interpersonal relationships and enhanced by an understanding of the factors affecting behavior.

General Behavioral Objective:

The student will be able to identify persons with whom feelings might be shared.

Domain: Affective   *Dimension:* Emotional

Grade Level: Upper elementary

Specific Behavioral Objective:

After identifying the emotions felt in selected situations, the student will be able to identify people with whom these feelings might be shared by completing a chart.

Directions: (Teacher)

    1. Duplicate the "Sharing Feelings is Important" worksheet (see p. 262).
    2. Read introduction to students.

Introduction:

Sometimes you have experiences that cause you to have strong feelings. When you feel this way, it is important that you share these feelings with someone you trust. Can you tell us why?

What might happen to someone who keeps his/her feelings all bottled up inside?

Suggested Follow-Up:

1. Use the words in the emotions list to make either
   a. a word-search puzzle, or
   b. a scrambled word puzzle
2. Use each of the emotion words in a sentence.

"SHARING FEELINGS IS IMPORTANT!"
WORKSHEET

Directions:

1. Here are some situations that might cause you to have strong feelings.
2. Read each situation carefully.
3. Choose one or more of the emotions you might feel from the list.
4. Write them in the space provided.
5. Decide with whom you would like to share these feelings. Write the names of these persons in the space provided.

EMOTIONS YOU MIGHT FEEL

angry/mad	love
afraid	shame
hate	joy
sad	stupid
lonely	clumsy
happy	worried
excited	frustrated
embarrassed	puzzled
jealous	depressed
proud	confused

SITUATION	FEELINGS	SHARE WITH WHOM?
1. Your pet dog has been killed by an automobile.		
2. You open your presents on Christmas morning.		
3. You are invited to your best friend's birthday party.		
4. You are sent to your room for punishment.		
5. Your mother got a promotion at work.		
6. Your father tells you how pleased he is that you are doing well in school.		
7. You are having trouble understanding the arithmetic lesson.		
8. You get blamed for something you didn't do.		
9. You did something you shouldn't have done. Your brother squeals on you.		
10. You tripped and fell and got a black eye.		

the joy of being creative

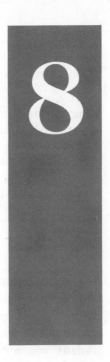

8

Ideas, Ideas, Ideas

The sale of recipe books is a big business in our country. People who are vitally interested in pursuing the culinary arts are constantly experimenting with new concoctions of foods. They want to add a variety of tastes, colors, nutrients, and other such qualities to spice up the menues to whet their own appetites and those of the people they serve. When neophytes begin to cook, they learn by communicating with and observing others doing their thing and by using basic recipe books that deal with the fundamentals of cooking. As experience is gained, they begin to branch out. And, always, good cooks put a bit of themselves—their own personality—into their every creation.

Can you see the analogy between becoming a better-than-average cook and becoming a better-than-average teacher? The same kind of experience holds true for teachers who are concerned with their own personal growth and effectiveness and who are sold on what they are selling. They learn by communicating, observing, and experimenting—and they make learning more palatable for their students and teaching more enjoyable for themselves.

ADAPTING OTHER'S IDEAS

It doesn't suffice, however, for teachers to take someone else's ideas and designs and use them exactly as prescribed. Good teachers use others' ideas and spice them up by redesigning them to meet their own needs and those of their students. And, always, they put a bit of their own personality and creativity into the pot.

To illustrate this concept, a small group of teachers in a survey were given this stem sentence to complete:

Recently, in a ——————— lesson, I had my kids . . . . and it really worked.

Here are just a few of the off-the-cuff replies that were submitted.

At the beginning of the year, in a science lesson I had my kids make a theater mask collage showing their likes and dislikes. This helped to give me initial insight into each child as a person. While my first goal was to get to know them, I was also able to discover how well each student was able to follow directions, properly use the materials, and who among them took pride in his/her work.[1]

Recently, in an English lesson when we were discussing personality, I had my kids outline each of their faces on a large sheet of plain, white paper. Using this color code, they were asked to cut out and paste on the eyes, mouth, nose, ears, etc. in the colors appropriate to demonstrate their own character traits in the face:

RED = fun-loving
BLUE = serious
GREEN = envious
YELLOW = kind
BLACK = sad
ORANGE = compassionate

The entire face had to be filled in so that no white showed. Upon completion, each student discussed his/her own face and explained why the colors were employed. These were then displayed throughout the room.[2]

---

[1] *Patricia J. Cermak, Middleburg Heights Jr. High School, By permission.*
[2] *Carolyn Kasler, Middleburg Heights Jr. High School, By permission.*

Recently, in a science lesson, in order to teach students the importance of procedure in carrying out experiments, I had my kids, in small groups, write up the step-by-step procedure for making a peanut butter-and-jelly sandwich. When they finished I collected them. Pretending to have literally no knowledge of procedure, I then attempted to make a sandwich following their directions. For instance, if their procedure did not call for opening the jar of peanut butter, I would not open it. If it directed me to insert the knife into the jar, I attempted to do it through the lid or the side of the jar. Some procedures may have asked me to turn the lid without mentioning that I needed to hold the jar at the same time. At any rate, following some of their procedures, it was impossible for me to make the sandwich.

The learning experience brings the point home that proper *procedure*, both in write-ups and experiments, are very important. What students *do* or *don't do* in conducting an experiment could result in injury, poor results, or having to repeat the entire procedure. This lesson was well-remembered. It worked![3]

DEVELOPING YOUR OWN IDEAS

The design ideas in Chapter 7 of this book were provided to serve as a springboard from which teachers can vault. The reader *must not* accept them as being complete learning in any concept. They are merely ideas of others that are intended to spark the imagination and creativity that are present in every facilitator. The kind of learning experiences that are provided only give examples that several individuals have designed. As you can see, there are no original methods utilized. The originality and creativity lies in the development of a behavioral objective that blends an existing method with a specific focus on a domain and a dimension. By melding the content to the concept, the designer succeeds in developing a different way of providing another opportunity for the students to use in developing a stated competency or ability.

When you read about, hear, or see the way someone else designs a learning experience and think, "That's a good idea, but it could be better if . . .", then you're on your way to developing *your own* ideas.

There are several excellent elementary health education textbook

[3] *Donald Masaitis, Middleburg Heights Jr. High School, By permission.*

series on the market today. Using these, other resource materials, and your own creativity in designing and redesigning, every classroom teacher can have meaningful health education in the classroom.

We're all in this business together to educate children better. It is *not* a sin to employ a variety of methods to reach the learning objectives. Rather it can be expected that learning will become a more enjoyable and meaningful experience for kids. They will experience growth in every dimension by . . . *Learning, Feeling,* and *Doing.*

putting points on the board

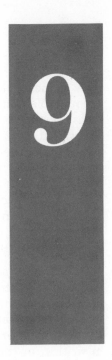

9

Accountability in the Classroom

As professional educators all of us want and need to score in the game. But as in any other contest there are always some frustrations to be encountered in achieving success. Whatever your teaching style is, the word "accountability" keeps appearing on the teaching scene. It isn't a word or a concept to be feared. Accountability is a reality of life in any job we tackle. We *need* to be accountable!

The word "accountability" has been used, misused, and abused in pedagogical language for many years. It has been interpreted to mean different things by different people, depending upon who is speaking or writing. The dictionary defines it as a "state of being accountable, liable, or responsible".[1] For teachers, the word basically asks three questions:

(1) Have my students *really* learned something?

(2) How do *they* know that they have learned?

(3) How do *I* know that they have learned?

In this book, the authors have attempted to encourage use of a

---

[1] By permission from Webster's Third New International Dictionary © 1976 by G & C Merriam Co., Publishers of the Merriam-Webster Dictionaries.

design model which should help teachers answer these questions and quell some of the fear they may have about proving themselves accountable. The model, if followed, provides the opportunity to measure student performance in the three domains of learning. Each assessment opportunity is structured into the behavioral objectives. After the concepts, toward which the learning will be aimed, have been selected, the general behavioral objectives formulated, and the specific, measurable objectives structured to accomplish the general behavioral objectives, the teacher will actually be able to observe whether the learning has indeed taken place.

SCORING IN THE ACCOUNTABILITY GAME

For some, accountability is limited to asking how many facts a student can recall in a testing situation. While "knowing" facts can be useful, we think that being able to "do" something as a result of knowing the facts is of even more importance. Thus, what has become a higher priority for us is such as being able to explain verbally, in writing, or through visual representation; to identify ways; and to express opinions based upon facts. We feel very strongly that we are being more accountable in helping our students develop ways to apply the facts in learning, to cope with the problems they face, or to manage their personal concerns than we would be if the "bottom line" were only a numerical grade based on recall of facts.

How do students know if they have learned? Probably the easiest way is for the teacher to share the objectives with them. They must be able to understand what is expected of them. If this is done, they too will be able to measure their own performance.

It is true that there are many factors affecting how much and how well students learn. Some can be controlled by the teacher, others cannot. Certainly it is beyond the teacher's realm or purpose to control students' biological capabilities or to alter the environments outside of the school in which they operate. However, every teacher *is* accountable, liable, and responsible for what takes place *in* the classroom — the kind of *nurturing opportunities* that are available to facilitate students' physical, mental, emotional, and social growth.

You're the pro! Go out and put more points on the board!

Index